"Next to telling her age, the most horrible mistake a woman can make is believing the golden promises in the cosmetic ads. . . .

"Americans spend $7 billion a year on what's loosely called 'grooming aids.' And having just cleaned out two medicine chests, a vanity table, a linen cupboard, and two bedside commodes, and discarded what looks like a million dollars' worth of cosmetics, I've come to the conclusion that we're all a pack of fools. . . .

"Cosmetically speaking, women were better off in the days when they brewed their own beauty aids."

—Harriet Van Horne
New York Post

HERE'S EGG ON YOUR FACE
Or How to Make Your Own Cosmetics
was originally published by
Hewitt House.

Here's Egg On Your Face

BEATRICE TRAVEN

with the assistance of

Dr. Ferenc Tibor

PUBLISHED BY POCKET BOOKS NEW YORK

HERE'S EGG ON YOUR FACE

OR HOW TO MAKE YOUR OWN COSMETICS

Hewitt House edition published June, 1970

Pocket Book edition published April, 1971

This *Pocket Book* edition includes every word
contained in the original, higher-priced edition. It is printed
from brand-new plates made from completely reset, clear, easy-to-read
type. *Pocket Book* editions are published by Pocket Books, a division
of Simon & Schuster, Inc., 630 Fifth Avenue, New York, N.Y. 10020.
Trademarks registered in the United States and other countries.

Standard Book Number: 671-77278-3.
Library of Congress Catalog Card Number 73-112452.

Printed in the U.S.A.

TO all the women in the world who ever held a mysterious cosmetic jar in their hands—and wished it weren't so mysterious.

PREFACE

What happens when a simple housewife, owner of the world's largest collection of half-used cosmetic jars and bottles, and a renowned cosmetic chemist, who formulated half the cosmetics that came in them, meet, talk, and decide to do a book together?

Why would they ever do a thing like that? Partly because the housewife—whom I hereby reveal to be me—found herself so fascinated by what the cosmetic chemist, Dr. Ferenc Tibor, revealed about beauty products: what they are and *aren't;* what they can and *can't* do; what they should and shouldn't be. Partly, I think, because Dr. Tibor, face to face with The Consumer (the anonymous Lady for whom he'd been compounding all his elegant jams and jellies for so many years) found out how little she really knows of what he does, or why—and how eager she is to learn. So many times she has trustingly expected miracles from her little pots of cream, spurred on, no doubt, by the airy puffery of the cosmetic ads. And so many, many times she's ended up by throwing or giving away a cream which, if she hadn't demanded the impossible, would have given her pleasure with its elegant texture, color, and fragrance, and helped her to keep her skin at its best with moisturizers, emollients, and conditioners—and, in short, completely fulfilled the function for which it was created.

But how's a girl to know what is and isn't possible, what's in beauty products, what each ingredient is there for, and which cosmetics are *right* for her and which aren't? Why, by making them herself, of course! We threw down the gauntlet to Dr. T. (who promptly recoiled in horror!). Why not a cosmetic cookbook, with recipes

7

("Formulas," said Dr. T.) *recipes*, that any woman could follow, using ingredients that women could understand, could *buy* in supermarkets, or drug stores, or the like— recipes that explained *how* and *why* cosmetic products worked or didn't? And what's more, how about recipes that we could *alter, play with,* as any creative cook does with the recipes she likes best, so that we could *custom-tailor* our cosmetics, make exactly what we liked best for the kind of skin or hair *we* were blessed with?

"Hmmm," said Dr. T.

And what's still more, how about using *fresh* ingredients, things that we could buy *today,* and use *now,* and keep refrigerated—things that cosmetic companies surely have to duplicate with chemicals because they can't afford the luxury of buying them fresh? At this point, Dr. T. looked definitely intrigued.

And so this cookbook was born. Every one of the recipes in it is original, formulated by Dr. T., tested by him in his wife's kitchen (and often the laboratory wizard burned his finger on the Pyrex cup) and pronounced by him equal to, or superior to, equivalent products selling on the market. What's more, every recipe offers many variations, so that the home cosmeticook who really learns her craft in these pages can go on to make many, many more products —the number limited only by her own imagination and the rate at which her family and friends can consume her creations!

It goes without saying that cosmeticookery is a good deal less costly than delicious indulgence in elegant store-bought products. For the amount you might pay for one super-luxurious eye cream, you can probably buy all the ingredients needed to make every recipe in this book. But a penny saved is by no means our main goal. Our hope is that learning to make your own cosmetics—learning the *reasons* why certain ingredients are used, the *rationale behind the mystique* of cosmetics—will not only make you a more intelligent consumer of those you *do* choose to buy, but also give you the delight of making the very product you'd like best, the thing you couldn't afford to have any cosmetic company formulate for you: the thing that's *just right for you.*

One housewife at least (again revealed to be me) enjoyed this pleasure, and learned, and learned, and learned. Dr. Tibor (nursing his burnt fingers) admits that he learned, too. By being forced back to simple natural ingredients (because that's all this housewife could buy) he had to improvise, be ingenious, confront on the ground floor the basic principles of his craft. He haunted the supermarkets for cosmetic bargains as eagerly as any bride, moaned and muttered over his failures, whooped and strutted over his successes. He came out of it all, he tells us, with increased understanding of cosmetic chemistry, and of the Lady, that hopeful demanding anonymous Lady for whom he has labored all these many years.

"I have met the enemy," he sighs with twinkly gallantry, "and I am theirs."

COMMON SENSE ABOUT SENSITIVITY

All cosmetics demand a certain amount of common sense in the using, and those you make yourself are no exception.

Though chances are that the recipes in this book are simpler, purer, and less irritating than most of what you buy and use, certain minimum precautions should be observed.

Before you use *any* cosmetic, bought or concocted, for the first time, it's only sensible to *try it out* on a bit of you that's highly sensitive. If it doesn't react there, it probably won't elsewhere. Rub a bit of *any* new cosmetic on the skin on the inside of your elbow, cover it with an adhesive bandage, and leave it on overnight. If there's no redness or reaction in the morning, you can be reasonably sure the cosmetic is fine for you. Naturally, if you use any beauty product and it makes you feel itchy, irritated, or in any way uncomfortable, you'd stop using it, and this is as true of those you cook up from these recipes as of any commercial ones you might buy.

There are those of you who know yourselves to be sensitive to certain ingredients (such as strawberries or eggs or nylon or wool fibers). You should be especially cautious in trying any new product that you might be sensitive to, and if you suspect that any beauty product is causing an unpleasant reaction, you should naturally discontinue its use immediately. For you, this book might have a special bonus: knowing what ingredients are unfriendly to you, you can try leaving them out, substituting around them, formulating your cosmetics in the way that is most comfortable for *you*.

And to be even more certain, if you know you have an allergy—or suspect you might have one—discuss these recipes with your doctor before you try any of them.

There are times when *all* of us are sensitive to things we might not normally react to—when our skin is irritated already, for instance, or when we're sunburned or chafed, or when the drying action of soaps or harsh materials have stripped away some of the normal protective mantle of the skin and left it without its natural complement of oils and sebum. At these times, we should be extra-careful to keep away from anything that's even slightly uncomfortable on our skin.

These are simple precepts. Most of us know and observe them in our everyday use of cosmetics and beauty products. They hold equally true for the recipes given here. There is one more *absolute rule:* never use *any* cosmetic on an already irritated skin; cosmetics are *not* drugs and should not be used as substitutes for doctors or medicines.

With these commonsense precautions in mind, dive in, cook away, and enjoy the great pleasure of creating and using some of the finest, most wholesome, most elegant cosmetics you'll ever dab a finger to!

CONTENTS

INTRODUCTION

If there is a single time-honored tradition in the annals of femininity, it is the practice of women making their own cosmetics. Cleopatra surely didn't stand over a firepot concocting her own beauty treatments, but she surely *did* depend on the kohl, ointments, unguents, and oils whipped up by some talented handmaiden. Old housewifery books, from the Middle Ages onward, abound with dark hints about magical beauty formulas, and by the time your grandma or mine was old enough to care about the whiteness of her skin and the pinkness of her nails, she knew enough to brew up herbal complexion vinegars, milks, toilet waters, pomades, buff-rouges, special soaps, shampoos, and what-have-you.

It's only in modern times, with such a bewildering (and seductive) variety of cosmetics available to us, and so much more money to spend on life's little niceties than ever before, that we women have lost the nerve or the knack of whipping up our little beauty jams and jellies ourselves. In so doing, we've relinquished the special pleasure of hand-making our beauty preparations to do exactly the job we want done. But even more of a loss, we've buried a whole carefully-handed-down education in what various creams and oils and fruit and vegetable juices and extracts and tinctures and teas and spirits and milk and butter and eggs can *do* for the skin.

Our grandmas knew. Our great-great-great grandmas knew. They cultivated herb gardens and treasured secret recipes and scorned "face paint" and cosseted their peach-fuzz petal-soft skin that didn't *need* face paint. They knew what natural products would gloss up their hair and soften their hands and whiten their teeth. And we, for the most part, *don't*. We educated moderns have really missed out on a lot!

For instance—what is it possible for a cosmetic to do? Obviously *no* beauty preparation, no matter how much you sigh and wish to the contrary, is going to iron out wrinkles, do miracles for large pores or pimples by making old skin young, or sensitive skin tough, or olive skin fair. (Which elicits a sigh from the dreamers; there was a time when you couldn't make curly hair straight, or straight hair curly, or brown hair blonde. Maybe *someday* . . . ?)

A cosmetic isn't a drug, and can't cure or prevent conditions which are in the province of doctors and prescriptions. They're not magic, and they're not medicine. All right, then (that established)—what *are* they?

First of all, a cosmetic should give *pleasure*. It should look and smell and feel delicious. It should offer a psychological lift to the person using it; making a cosmetic is truly making a gift—for yourself, or whoever you offer it to. And like a gift, it should be very special, very carefully chosen by the giver for the receiver (most especially if both of them are *you*).

Second of all, a cosmetic enhances the appearance of whatever part of you it's meant for. It might help gloss or condition your hair, body it or make it more manageable, help you to set or slick it down. A cosmetic might help give an oily skin a drier look, or a dry one a dewier glow. It might soften the appearance of wrinkles on face or hands, stimulate the skin a bit to make it blushy, protect it with a thin film of cream against the wear and tear of sun, soap, salt water, or the drying of central heating. It might cover or color your skin, if it's a makeup, cool and refresh you, cleanse you, smooth down itchy dry skin scales, bathe you, powder you—in all ways work to make you more comfortable and more beautiful.

Third, if you do *faithfully* use the right beauty products for you, over the long haul you can and will keep your skin beautifully clean, and more supple, fresh and young-looking than if you'd simply abandoned it to what time, neglect, and exposure can do. Careful, sensible skin pampering pays off—and if you don't believe it, look at the difference between a farm woman of forty who's washed her face with soap and water all her life, been exposed to sun and wind daily, and would no more cream her hands, face and throat than she would dance in her nightie—and any bright suburban housewife or career gal of forty who's wise to the ways of cosmetics and doesn't think it's pampering to enjoy what God gave her and keep it as long and as well as possible. You'd never, never mistake one for the other. Convinced?

Here's egg on your face!

CHAPTER ONE

TOOLS OF THE TRADE

First, since all of the ingredients we're using can be washed off with sufficient hot water, soap, and elbow grease, you needn't be afraid to use any kitchen tools you have on hand. Some of the ingredients, like hard waxes (beeswax, paraffin), and certain fats (like lanolin) leave a film on pans or containers that is *difficult* to remove. So for these items only, it's advisable to keep special containers—like old baby food jars or small tin cans—reserved exclusively for them. Make sure to *label* these containers carefully! Then when you need some beeswax, or some lanolin, you can just take out the jarful, place it over boiling water to melt it, pour off what you need, and let the rest reharden.

The very minimum you'll need for your cosmeticookery is as follows:

one or two eyedroppers: for measuring food color, perfumes, or for making tests of small amounts of oils or lotions. You can get these at your drug store or wash out old ones from eye drops.

one or two thin blade spatulas: called "palette knives," available in art supply stores, or you may already have one among your kitchen stuff. The best length is about four-to-five inches, and the spatula should be quite flexible. The blade should be stainless steel. You will be using these for hand mixing of small (one cup or less) quantities of cream, to scrape out creams from making-pot to jar, and to smooth down surfaces of jars. If you have both, you can substitute a knife and a rubber (not plastic) scraper for the versatile spatula.

19

a three-speed electric hand mixer: although you can do without it, your life will be much simplified, and your results generally much better *with* this handy tool. Even if you have the big-scale mixer, the *portable* kind is so versatile, mobile and light that it's worth considering. When making these recipes, use only *one* beater, except for very large batches. That way you can work in measuring cups, small pots, even in jars, and control small batches exceedingly well.

set of metal measuring spoons: don't use plastic, as it's likely to melt in your bubbling brews. Have you ever found yourself stirring with the *handle* of a plastic spoon? I have, and I don't recommend it to you!

one or two inexpensive enamel pots: you can buy them in the five-and-ten. If you're buying two, make one about two cup, the other about a quart. You want enamel rather than aluminum or anything else because it doesn't react with anything used in the recipes, and is relatively cheap. Glass is fine, too, and you could substitute for these a two-cup and a quart *Pyrex* glass measuring cup. (Be careful of the handles, though; they get *hot!*) If you have, or can afford, a double boiler, that's useful. If not—or maybe even if you can—try out the *wide flat pan* method of heating over boiling water, described below. It has one distinct advantage: two pots can be heating at the same time in the same water, so they reach about the same temperature together—and that's important when you form emulsions because the oil and water phases generally combine more cheerfully when they're at the same temperature.

one or two Pyrex measuring cups: if two, see above. If one, make it a two-cup on which the ounces are clearly marked.

containers: pester everybody for pretty jars and bottles (preferably with lids), and clean out and save the ones you buy. But if you have nothing elegant, save baby food jars, peanut butter jars, medicine bottles, so that you gradually build up a collection of varying sizes, with varying neck widths. Some drug stores will sell you jars and bottles, but again, beware of plastic! If it's not *dishwater* or *boil-proof,* it's not for you. A small funnel or bulb baster for getting those precious ingredients in small topped containers is a good idea.

labels: buy press-on or stick-on types at your stationery store, or, if you must, use a grease pencil. But never, *never* leave a jar unlabeled. Nobody's memory holds too well after a month or two, and it's a shame to end up throwing away an elegant cream because you can't remember which part of you it's for. If you *really* want to do things right, do what Dr. T. does: buy a notebook and keep track of *all* your cosmeti-cookery—date made, observations, ingredients, variations, results. It's fun, informative, and *very* good practice.

the wide low pan: Dr. T. used an electric fry pan for this, but you can use anything you have that will hold a couple of inches of water and two small pots and sit comfortably *(non-tippily)* on your kitchen range. If you have double boilers, you can use them in place of the wide, low pan, but our experiments were all carried on in the w.l.p. and we never had a miss in terms of temperatures, burns, spills, or boilovers. So we recommend it. In any case, anywhere we say "heat over boiling water," what we mean is, set your pot or measuring cup in the wide low pan full of boiling water and let it heat slowly (never heat fats or oils or waxes on direct heat!) until you've got it where we want it. So much for the wide low pan.

And that's all.

CHAPTER TWO

TRICKS OF THE TRADE

PLEASE READ THIS SECTION BEFORE YOU DO ANOTHER THING!

Eager cooks being what they are, you've probably already gotten out your measuring spoons and hefted your electric mixer. *Stop!* There are a few tricks of the trade, trade secrets, and just plain commonsense techniques that will save you worlds of time and guarantee superior results. Here they are. Study them, please, before you go one step further!

1. *Always read a recipe through* before beginning to work on it. Make sure you understand what's going to happen, how long it's likely to take, what size jars or bottles you'll need, what tools should be handy. It's *awful* to be nursing a delicate emulsion along, be ready to pour it out, and suddenly discover that there's nothing to pour it *into*. Don't let this happen to you! Be *sure* to look up *all* the ingredients in the INGREDIENTS section, and make sure you understand what's needed and, if you're substituting, what's possible and impossible.

2. *Be exact* in your measurements, and follow directions *precisely*. Dr. T. is a chemist, a scientist, and very picky. When he says one-fourth teaspoon he doesn't mean one-half teaspoon. And he means *level* measurements, except when he specifies otherwise. In cooking, you can put in a dib more of this and a dab less of that and still get good results. But these recipes are scientifically worked out, and failures can follow careless measuring or sloppy heating or

cooling techniques. To facilitate *precise measuring*, get in the habit of "rinsing off" the spoons you use to measure hard waxes in the hot oil called for in the recipe. That way you can be sure you've got every bit of wax. Do the same for fats that stick to the spoon. Another trick is to preheat your measuring spoon before you use it by holding it under hot water for a minute or two; then wipe it on a tissue and dip out your wax or fat, which will slip much more easily *off* a hot spoon than a cold one.

3. *Use wax base where possible* since various waxes that we use (beeswax, paraffin, stearic acid), are so hard. (*See* Base Stocks.) The *wax bases* are half wax, half oil, and therefore much softer and easier to melt and measure out than plain wax. Another trick for hard waxes is to melt some beeswax or paraffin, measure out some tablespoonful size dollops of it, pour each into an aluminum foil "cup" which you can make yourself by forming the foil around your thumb, then—when it's cool enough to handle—form each dollop into a ball, jar the balls (label them, please!), keep them in a cool place, and pop them into the pot with the other ingredients whenever your recipe calls for a tablespoon of wax. Easy?

4. *Watch your temperatures!* Creams and lotions are testy creatures. Both the oil and water phases should usually be at the same temperature when you mix them. Many emulsions will separate if they're kept too hot for too long; therefore pay careful attention to jar-ing or bottling instructions, and don't close the lid on them *hot* if they're supposed to *cool* first. Never freeze an emulsion; it will "break." (If you don't believe it, freeze a bit of non-homogenized milk—an oil/water emulsion of butterfat in water). So don't plan to make and freeze large batches of cosmetics, as you would stew or vegetable soup. If you want to make large quantities, see A Note About Preservatives. Emulsions enjoy cooling *gradually,* and being stirred more or less constantly as they cool. You can use your electric beater when the mixture is still hot and liquidy and the air bubbles can still escape. As it thickens, you'll

probably have to switch to hand mixing. *Some* of the recipes, on the other hand, call for "whipping" as the mixture cools down; this gives a lighter, better homogenized cream, a fluffy effect. Some creams go grainy if they are not properly mixed or beaten, so here, too, be sure to follow directions *exactly*. Never add perfume, flavor extracts, witch hazel or alcohol to your mixture while it's too hot, or they'll simply evaporate. Make sure you put these ingredients in only towards the end, when the pot is warm to the touch.

5. *Be sure each phase of an emulsion is thoroughly dissolved* and/or melted before you do the mix. If either phase has lumps in it, the result won't be right. Some of the Base Stocks are fairly thick or stiff. If you have any trouble dissolving them into a recipe, heat them gently as necessary until smooth.

6. *There may be times when something unavoidable* calls you away from your cosmeticooking, and pots warm too long or stand open and lose liquid. If this happens, try adding a tablespoon or so of warm water to the mix to make up for what's lost. Do it a tiny bit at a time, and watch carefully to make sure the batch accepts each bit. Mother your mixes and baby them; the care will pay lovely dividends later.

7. *In jar-ing or bottling, make sure that the containers you use are close to the size of your batch, boil-proof,* and *glass or metal* (*not* plastic). Too much air in a jar causes the product to go bad sooner than it would if less of it came in contact with the air. Similarly, trying to avoid air bubbles when scooping your creams into jars will protect them from going bad longer. Plastic is non grata because it so often isn't boil-proof, but also because certain oils and fats react with it, or even *permeate* it. As for metal, tin cans are fine, but stay away from copper, silver, brass, or any metal which reacts (rusts or corrodes) as it may spoil your delicate product.

8. *Never use direct heat,* unless specifically directed to. Oils and fats can burn very easily, and leave unpleasant odors and ugly discoloration in your final product. Overheating can even change the properties of a fat so that it won't emulsify properly. SOAP STOCK and other mixtures tend to foam up and over when heated directly on the stove burner. The best method is to use a *wide low pan,* like a large frying pan, baking pan, or electric fry pan, put a few inches of water in it, and heat *it* on your stove (or in the case of the fry pan, electrically). You can then place your pots, measuring cups or cans in the water to be heated; everything will move along more or less together, and you can pop things in and out at will. In the absence of a *wide low pan,* you can use one (or two, if you have them) double boiler(s), but all our experiments were carried out with the *w.l.p.,* and Dr. T. swears by it, so it remains far and away our first choice.

9. *You can often cool* your jar of cream or fat or whatever by putting it into a wide low pan of cold water, even with a few ice cubes floating in it. Don't put ice cubes into your batch, however, as they would dilute it, and cause local chilling, which is bad. Whenever chilling *or* heating, stir carefully, scraping down the sides of the container, so the whole mixture changes temperature at a steady, even rate. This is especially important in quick chilling, as otherwise solid cream forms at the sides and makes lumps while the center of the mix is still liquid.

10. *Always use Pyrex or metal* (see number seven for what kinds of metal to avoid) for cooling or warming, and never subject glass to extremes of hot and cold. When warming jars, start them in tepid water, and heat *gradually;* the same is true, in reverse, for cooling. Otherwise— cold jar in boiling water = cra-A-A-A-CK!

11. *When cleaning up,* don't try to wash large globs of cream or fat from utensils. *Wipe off* with a paper towel first, then use *very hot* running water to melt off most of the rest, and finally, wash with plain soap and warm water.

CHAPTER THREE

A NOTE ABOUT
PRESERVATIVES

None of the recipes in this book contain *added* preservatives. A few do contain natural preservatives, such as alcohol.

In general, therefore, you should treat these products as you would natural foods. They *will* tend to spoil eventually, especially those that contain a large percentage of water, on which most bacteria grow. Most of the creams will keep a month or two without problems, often much longer. *All of them will do better if kept tightly capped.* Once you open them, there's more chance that they may spoil and develop a musty or rancid odor.

There are several ways of avoiding this. First, of course, is to make only small batches and use them *fresh.* Since one of the main purposes of this book is to give you the luxury of *fresh* cosmetics, we've purposely kept the amounts of the recipes down to around a cupful, and we encourage you to make small batches and use them up or give them as presents so you *can* have the benefits of freshly made products.

Secondly, you can simply keep your products in the refrigerator—*not* the freezer, which will break most emulsions.

Third, you *can* add preservatives, as every manufacturer of commercial cosmetics does. Unfortunately you can't get hold of some of the best preservatives used for this purpose, but there are quite a few that *are* available to you. *However,* you should be aware that some preservatives— like some perfumes, by the way—can cause separation of your cream or lotion. Therefore, you should make up the recipe first; modify it to your own taste, learning the proper procedure by heart. *Then,* if you like it enough to want a lot of it around, and find it doesn't keep well—*then* try *adding* one of the following preservatives:

For acid preparations (such as those containing lemon juice): dissolve a pinch of salicylic acid or sodium benzoate in the oil phase.

For alkaline preparations (containing borax, or SOAP STOCK): add a few drops of merthiolate, or a few drops of tincture of iodine, white or brown.

For mostly water or water/alcohol preparations with low alcohol content: add a pinch of boric acid powder.

For any preparation to be used near the eyes: use nothing but a pinch of boric acid.

CHAPTER FOUR

ABOUT PERFUMES

Perfumes are pure luxury—they don't have a sensible function in the world except to delight you and make you beg for more. How marvellous!

One old advertisement for the original Eau de Cologne, printed in 1747, claimed it was:

> ... a volatile spirit, extracted from rare herbs and the most exquisite; from this is formed an elixir which has the property of restoring those parts of the body attacked by all manner of diseases. A moderate and lively warmth is imparted which, in sympathy with that of the patient, revives the vital spirits.

A wild exaggeration. *All* fragrances are primarily compounded to give pleasure, pure and simple. And they do. That's why no self-respecting cosmetic would be without one.

The ancients knew how to extract fragrance, distill it, preserve it. Their methods are well known and are still practiced to some extent to obtain the finest perfume ingredients today. Yes, we have giant modern stills and synthetic ingredients to lower the cost—and cheapen the fragrance—of many of the perfumes on the market. But you can still *do it yourself* in the old way, and get great pleasure, and a superior product, with very little trouble. Here's how:

Gather your flowers with as little stalk as possible, and put them into a jar filled with a bland oil (like olive oil or sweet almond oil). Melted lard can also be used or shortening (hydrogenated, for cooking, which is very well preserved and not likely to get rancid and odorous), or use *any* fat which is essentially odorless and mild.

Let the flowers stand in the oil for twenty-four hours, to extract the fragrance. Then filter off the blossoms through a coarse cloth, warming the fat slightly to remelt it if you've used a solid one. Throw away the spent flowers and repeat the process with fresh blossoms three or four times, thus gradually increasing the strength of your perfume to the point desired.

When you've reached the strength you like, mix your fragrant fat with an equal amount of 70 percent *ethanol* rubbing alcohol (*not* isopropyl). Put the fat-alcohol mixture in a tightly closed bottle, and shake vigorously. Let it stand a day. Shake again, daily, this way for at least a week. Then let the fat and alcohol separate, pour off the now-fragrant spirits of alcohol, and there it is—your own perfume!

(Note that the remaining oil will still be fragrant, so don't throw it away! *Use it.* Put it into some of the recipes in this book, substituting part or all of this fragrant oil for any *other* oil, and thus perfume your cosmetics with your own home-brewed fragrance, perhaps your favorite rose or carnation.)

Note, too, that you don't have to extract the essential oils from your fat at all. You can simply strain it very carefully until it is quite clear, and use it as is—in a bath oil, as a sachet for lockets, or whatever.

In this form, before extraction, solid fats *with fragrance* are called "concretes"—and certain concretes of such rare fragrances as rose or jasmine bring a very high price (up to hundreds of dollars per pound) and are eagerly sought by the finest perfume houses.

This process of absorbing the natural flower fragrances into solid fats is called "enfleurage," and—in this simple home version—will produce beautiful perfumes which, however, may prove to be somewhat short-lived, especially when they're extracted into alcohol. That's because you don't have available the various fixatives, rare natural substances like ambergris from the whale or civet from the wild civet cat of Ethiopia, that the perfume industry uses to fix fragrances. However, *any* fat or oil helps to hold fragrance to some degree, so keep your own concretes, and *use* them.

Another way to make your own perfumes is to extract the fragrance of dried herbs or tobacco directly into alcohol. To do this, "wet out" as many leaves as will comfortably fit in a bottle filled with 70 percent *ethanol* alcohol, let stand a day or two, strain the leaves off, and refill the alcohol with more leaves. Repeat this process several times until the alcohol is strongly colored and very fragrant. Then use it for part or all of the perfume called for. You can be wildly ingenious in the herbs you use—and combine. A few *we* especially like are tarragon, bay leaves, rosemary, mint, fennel seeds, anis, cardamom, thyme, vanilla beans, cloves, mace, nutmeg, ginger, basil, lemon peel, and cumin. Mix your own!

Your drugstore will also be the source of some elegant fragrances. Try asking for rose geranium oil, rose soluble oil, spirits of peppermint, lavender, bay rum, oil of cloves, or whatever else your druggist—who by now should be intrigued—has to suggest. All of the above are fairly inexpensive, and can be bought in minute quantities, which is all you'll need.

Just remember that extracts, tinctures, and the like—alcohol-based fragrances—are what you'll use in products that have alcohol as a major ingredient, and the fragrant fats and true perfume oils can be used only in products where fats or oils are major ingredients.

Be creative, and joyous, and enjoy! Happy sniffing.

CHAPTER FIVE

FRAGRANCE PRODUCTS

Men's after shaves, men's colognes, women's splash colognes and after bath coolers are all based on the same principle—a *good* fragrance, suitable for the particular use for which it's intended (and yes, there *are* men's and women's fragrances); include the correct *amount* of the fragrance (after shaves contain the least, colognes about twice as much, toilet waters double that again, and perfumes about double *that)* dissolved in a high alcohol base. to give lift to the fragrance and a cool feeling on the skin.

In the case of after shaves, which are splashed on over occasional razor nicks, the alcohol level can't be too high. Most men like a little "zing" in their after shave, without too much "ouch!" So most commercial after shaves are about 50 to 65 percent alcohol, plus a bit of perfume and some skin conditioners and emollients. "Low sting" after shaves sometimes dip down to as little as 35 percent alcohol, with a corresponding jump in skin conditioners—thereby substituting *cling* for *zing.*

When you concoct these products for your favorite man, feel free to improvise. Give him the amount of tingle he likes best, his favorite fragrance, and a color that suggests maleness or tingle or coolth—whatever seems most appropriate. It's the *tinkering,* the creativity with which you tackle home cosmetics, that really makes the difference between simply following the recipe—which will give you a fine product, equal or better to most of what you can buy on the market—and *custom tailoring* your products to suit the exact fancy of the specific person for whom they're intended. And cosmetics, after all, are a delicious luxury, an extra. So go to it, and make them special!

The same basic formulas that give you after shaves will also, with a little adjustment of color and scent, make gorgeous splash colognes, friction rubs, and misty after bath lotions. They're easy to make, can be beautifully colored and perfumed, and, because the ingredients are so inexpensive, you can splash them on with abandon.

There *is* one small problem, dear home cosmetic chemist, in making *all* these fragrance products—and this demands a little ingenuity. The basic procedure is simplicity itself: just dissolve all the ingredients in alcohol plus water, age a few days, then filter to get bright clarity. The problem is that practically none of the emollients available to you are either water or alcohol soluble! Dozens are available to commercial formulators; in fact the manufacture of emollients specifically for this purpose is big business, with many millions of gallons sold each year. But working solely out of the drug store and the supermarket, we had to be ingenious and find emollients which *would* dissolve, so the recipes which follow may strike you as a little different in appearance or skin feel from the products you're used to buying. You may have to talk your man into shaking his after shave before he puts it on, or into using less than usual in some cases to avoid a slight tackiness. But they are all eminently usable, and pleasant, and fun, and surprisingly easy to make. So concoct away. And don't be afraid of perfumes. (Read About Perfumes, chapter 4, and dare to dream up your own!) Remember—more perfume oil is used each year in the U.S. for men's cosmetic products (primarily after shaves) than for women's. And the trend is *up!*

SUPERSIMPLE GLYCERINE AND ROSEWATER

> 1 tbsp. witch hazel
> 2 tbsp. glycerine
> ¼ cup plus 1 tbsp. water
> ½ tsp. rose soluble perfume oil

Combine ingredients, stir together, and bottle. Presto— you're a cosmetic chemist!

Well, not quite. But you *have* concocted—and improved upon—one of the oldest and simplest of home cosmetics.

Your mama and mine used glycerine-rosewater in a variety of ways: on chapped lips or to ward them off, to soften calluses or rough elbows and heels, on dishpan hands, or as a general moisturizer on face and skin.

The classical glycerine-rosewater recipe called for a 50–50 mixture of each, *period*. Sometimes the rosewater was made at home, by steeping the petals. But nowadays most drug stores stock a "rose soluble" perfume oil which you can simply add to water in the strength you like. (One-half teaspoon is what *Dr. T.* likes, but you can experiment with from one-third to two-thirds teaspoon—twenty to forty drops—and choose the amount that suits your fancy, and your nose!) Probably the same drugstore will also carry a rosewater solution already made up, or even glycerine-rosewater itself, in the old 50–50 combination.

But in this day and age ladies like their cosmetics to be elegant, not sticky or tacky, and the 50–50 old faithful has too much glycerine to measure up to these standards.

So—our cosmetic chemist recommends cutting the classic version with an equal amount of water (thereby getting a 25–75 mixture) or—much more creative—using the SUPERSIMPLE, but artful, variation described.

SUPERSIMPLE G-R GEL

½ cup SUPERSIMPLE GLYCERINE AND ROSEWATER
2–4 tsp. dry gum tragacanth (or gum arabic)

Add the dry gum to the glycerine-rosewater and stir thoroughly. Let stand overnight, shaking occasionally for the first hour or two, so that the gum goes into solution.

The next day, if your gel has not formed, warm the solution slowly, stirring constantly to be sure *all* the gum has dissolved. Let cool. If it's still not thick enough to please you—it should be like beautiful, soft, clear gelatine dessert—just add a little more gum and repeat the procedure.

If you live in a small town, gum trag or gum arabic may be a little hard to track down. Art or ceramic supply stores stock it as a fixative for pastels and charcoal drawings, or as an ingredient to improve the texture of glazes and slip. (Do *not* buy the thin spraying solutions of gum trag which are occasionally offered by art supply stores; these are much too weak for cosmetic purposes.) Botanical stores stock dry gum trag, and so do some (old-fashioned) drugstores. Most could order it for you from *their* suppliers. If you have a choice, get it as "ribbons" rather than as dry powder; the ribbon form dissolves much more readily.

If you absolutely *can't* find either gum trag or gum arabic—or if you're stuck in the house and can't get out to try—you might experiment with cornstarch, boiling up two teaspoons of cornstarch with two tablespoons of glycerine plus one-half cup water, then, when it thickens, cooling it a bit and adding the amount of rose soluble perfume you favor, and letting the whole batch cool. It should gel nicely into a good substitute for the original SUPERSIMPLE.

BASIC AFTER SHAVE

1 tsp. glycerine
4 tbsp. witch hazel
¾ cup 70% *ethanol* rubbing alcohol
1 tsp. almond extract
1 tsp. anise extract
1 tsp. vanilla extract
1 tsp. peppermint extract

Simply mix all ingredients together, strain through an old (clean!) nylon stocking, and bottle. Makes about one cup.

If you don't wear nylons, or have no old ones on hand, don't despair. Line a fine strainer with paper towels and carefully pour your after shave through. Presto, it's filtered!

(For ultimate clarity of the product—a "polish filter" in

the parlance of the trade—let your after shave *stand one week,* then pour through paper towels. The main disadvantage of the paper towel over the nylon stocking technique is that you blot up some of your precious concoction.)

This makes a sparkling, invigorating after shave without a hint of tackiness. You can go creative by adding a few drops of food coloring (we like green or blue) or by substituting any other perfume or flavoring extracts you like for the almond, anise, and vanilla. Rum, brandy, or maple extracts are fun, or you can surprise your man by soaking his favorite brand of tobacco in alcohol (about one-third leaves to two-thirds alcohol; steep for about a week, then strain and use as custom scent). Probably you'll want to use a few drops of vanilla, too, to round off the scent, but go easy—it also adds sweetness. Don't leave out the peppermint, though; its contribution is the cooling *menthol* sensation. Another intriguing scent for after shave is tarragon. Steep it and strain it just as you would tobacco (above), changing the leaves several times during the week for extra strength. You'll either love it or loathe it—but nobody will guess it!

VELVET AFTER SHAVE

2 tsp. glycerine
½ tsp. boric acid powder
¼ cup plus 2 tbsp. witch hazel
½ cup plus 2 tbsp. 70% *ethanol* rubbing alcohol
1 tsp. peppermint extract
⅓ tsp. tincture of benzoin
6 shakes aromatic bitters

Simply mix together, let stand, filter, and bottle, as BASIC AFTER SHAVE. Makes about one cup.

This slightly more complicated version of BASIC has a lovely amber color, is clear, smooth, and has a slight tightening feel. If you'd like to experiment, try a drop or two of food coloring—maybe green and blue—to make it look as well as feel cool.

Tincture of benzoin is an old-timey inhalant your mama used in vaporizers to clear your head and chest when you had the sniffles. When dabbed on the skin, however, it adds a tightening quality. The aromatic bitters, which you'll find in your supermarket or liquor store, is used here for its fragrance—deliciously warm and pungent. When you reach for the bitters, you might like to cut loose and add twenty drops of gin essence as well. (Dr. T. did, and got a truly sophisticated fragrance!)

SATIN SPLASH COLOGNE

    1 egg
    1 tbsp. glycerine
    1 tbsp. castor oil
    1 tbsp. witch hazel
    1 cup of 70% *ethanol* rubbing
       alcohol
    1 tsp. lemon extract
    ½ tsp. anise extract
    ½ tsp. peppermint extract
    1 drop food coloring

Separate egg and add the yolk to the glycerine and castor oil. (The egg white is lovely for masks, as you will eventually discover, so don't throw it away; refrigerate it and read on!) Stir together vigorously by hand with a whisk or fork, or single beater on your electric mixer (*low* speed). You have now created LECITHIN BASE, or MOTHER BASE #1. (*See* Base Stocks and Mother Bases.)

Add the witch hazel, and beat again until smooth.

Take *one teaspoon only* of this mixture, and add it to the ethanol alcohol. Add lemon, peppermint and anise extracts, plus the food coloring (green or red are lovely). Beat together thoroughly with your electric beater on *medium.* Makes about one cup.

SATIN SPLASH COLOGNE has an opaque, tingly fragrance

and a marvellous smooth skin feel. Use it after your bath—
or make some up for your husband; call it LUXURY AFTER
SHAVE, and see how pleased he'll be. (Splash colognes and
after shaves have virtually identical formulas.)

Are you surprised at the use of castor oil in this recipe?
It has several very special cosmetic qualities: it is partially
alcohol soluble (most oils aren't), is loaded with polyunsaturates (terrific for the skin), and leaves an especially
rich skin feel. And don't worry about the egg yolk going
bad; the alcohol will preserve it.

As for the LECITHIN BASE, or LECITHIN BASE-plus-witch-
hazel—this is the conditioning agent or heart of the formula, and as such is useful in a variety of ways. Used alone
on the skin it is a rich, rich conditioner. Added to simple
formulas, such as rosewater-glycerine or basic shampoos,
it conditions up a storm. So save what you have left over,
and experiment.

Label: Shake Before Using.

EMOLLIENT COLOGNE

> 2 tbsp. LECITHIN BASE (*see* Base
>   Stocks and Mother Bases)
> > *or*
>
> 1 egg
> 1 tbsp. glycerine
> 1 tbsp. castor oil

and

> 1 tbsp. witch hazel, *plus*
> ½ cup witch hazel
> ¼ cup 70% *ethanol* rubbing alcohol
> 1 drop food coloring
> ¼ tsp. rose soluble perfume oil

Separate egg and mix one tablespoon egg yolk with

glycerine, castor oil, and one tablespoon witch hazel. If you still have LECITHIN BASE left from SATIN SPLASH CO-LOGNE, or any other recipe, simply mix two tablespoons of the Base with one tablespoon witch hazel. Stir until smooth.

Now add the balance of the witch hazel and the alcohol, plus food coloring and perfume. Presto, a fragrant, gentle emollient cologne for after bath luxury. This recipe, too, can be used as well as an after shave—especially if your man has supersensitive skin.

The LECITHIN BASE in *this* cologne forms a stable dispersion (droplets suspended, not dissolved, therefore opaque) that doesn't need to be shaken before using. It's milder (less alcohol, more witch hazel), has less bite than an after shave; therefore it's a perfect conditioner for the man who really doesn't *like* zing and prefers emollients and protection against the drying effects of wind and sun.

The rose scent is very suave, but if you prefer, try mixing your own, aiming always to match silky feel with silky scent. (The low alcohol content in this product means you may have trouble getting perfume oils to stay in. They may tend to float up and require a light shaking before use.)

Another idea is to try and use two tablespoons of your favorite splash or friction cologne in place of two table-spoons of the alcohol in this recipe. This will scent the product and give a slightly different skin conditioning emolliency.

CHAPTER SIX

REFRESHERS

PINK PEARL SKIN FRESHENER

    2 tbsp. 70% *ethanol* rubbing
        alcohol
    ¼ cup plus 2 tbsp. water
    ¼ cup rosewater
    1 drop red food color
    ½ tsp. borax

(If you have rose soluble perfume oil on hand, substitute for the *water* and *rosewater,* one-half cup plus two tablespoons water plus ten drops rose perfume.)

Measure all ingredients into a large bottle (ten ounces is about right) and shake until thoroughly dissolved. Makes a bit over one cup.

Skin fresheners have a twofold purpose. They're coolly refreshing on a hot summer day—a sort of face splash cologne that's not drying, because of the low percentage of alcohol. Their other, and far more popular, use is as a follow-up to cleansing cream. The best cleansing creams are invariably oily, but having removed your makeup with an oily cream you then, paradoxically, want to remove the remover! Ergo, a *mild* skin freshener will do the trick and give your skin that dewy look and touch that makes it ready for bed—or another application of war paint.

For maximum results, *pat* on skin fresheners! Slap your cheeks gently to get the circulation going, working upward lightly with two pads of cotton wrung out in icy water and then saturated with PINK PEARL. Start at the base of your throat and pat, pat, pat right up to your forehead. Or keep PINK PEARL in the refrigerator and pat it on straight. Either way, it will leave you blushing and glowing—and ready for anything!

ASTRINGENT SKIN FRESHENER

- ¼ cup 70% *ethanol* rubbing alcohol
- ¼ cup water
- ⅓ cup orange flower water
- ⅓ cup rosewater
- ¼ tsp. powdered alum

Mix all the ingredients together, shake well, and bottle. Makes a bit over a cup.

If you can't get orange flower water for this recipe (and it's a pity if your druggist won't dig up some for you!) try substituting witch hazel plus one-fourth teaspoon lemon extract, or any other perfume oil. You can, of course, use a whole two-thirds cup of rosewater and go all the way with rose scent, which is lovely too.

In any case, this SKIN FRESHENER is mildly astringent, sparkling clear, and very refreshing. Because of the alum and high alcohol content, it's not recommended for make-up removal.

(BASIC types, such as PINK PEARL, with its bit of borax, do a better job of removing facial creams.) But ASTRINGENT is a wonder for oily skins, especially on humid summer days, when a brisk, toning facial pickup is just what you crave.

HERBAL ASTRINGENT

- ¼ cup tarragon extract (homemade)
- ¼ tsp. tincture of benzoin
- 1 tsp. glycerine
- ¼ tsp. boric acid powder
- 3 tbsp. witch hazel

First make the tarragon extract lovingly in advance, by soaking as many leaves of dried tarragon as you can comfortably wet out in a covered jar containing one-half cup of 70 percent *ethanol* alcohol. Don't jam the leaves in, but don't leave any "spaces" in the alcohol, either. After about a week of soaking, strain the leaves out through cheesecloth, and fill up your alcohol with another batch of dried leaves. Continue the process until a good strong fragrance and a rich *dark* olive color are obtained. (Needless to say, you can use *any* herb to make an *extract* or *tincture* in this way, or even tobacco leaves, if their smell intrigues you.)

Once you have your tincture of tarragon, dissolve the boric acid in the witch hazel, warming *slightly* if necessary. Do not overheat, or you'll lose the alcohol content of the witch hazel.

Add the glycerine to your tarragon extract, and stir until dissolved. Then add the tincture of benzoin and the witch hazel (boric acid solution). Stir thoroughly and bottle. Do *not* add perfume or coloring in this case, as both are handsomely supplied by the tarragon. Makes one-half cup of delicious green herbal astringent which you should apply sparingly, as a special treat.

An astringent generally is used to give tone to the skin; it has a cooling, firming, pore-tightening feel. If you like mild HERBAL ASTRINGENT, and want to try for more of the same, put together a bottle of more powerful—and more drying—PEPPERMINT PAT-ON.

PEPPERMINT PAT-ON ASTRINGENT

¾ cup of 70% *ethanol* rubbing alcohol
½ tsp. peppermint extract
¼ cup fresh lemon juice (reconstituted will work too, but fresh is *better*)
1 drop green food color

After you've squeezed your lemon juice (you'll need about one and one-half lemons), filter it carefully through paper towels laid over a strainer (unless you think you'd *like* the sensation of squishy pulp rubbed crispily against your skin—and why not, after all?—in which case, leave it virginal). Add the lemon juice to the rest of the ingredients; let stand until thoroughly settled, then filter again (or don't, in which case the lemon pulp will separate out and have to be shaken up before application each time). Bottle. Makes one cup of really zingy, mint-green astringent.

PEPPERMINT PAT-ON has everything: a whacking load of alcohol to serve up that tingle-and-glow sensation, a good shot of menthol (peppermint oil, which is dissolved in alcohol to make the peppermint extract sold in supermarkets, contains about 28 percent menthol) to add that icy coolth, and lemon juice to acidify your skin and give your pores an extra tightening. If you really want the ultimate in zinginess, try adding a pinch of alum (that's what styptic pencils are made of) to either of the above astringents. That'll give super-zing. (Not recommended for sissies!)

CHAPTER SEVEN

MASKS: WHAT THEY DO, WHAT THEY DON'T

Masks are for fun, for the imagination to go wild, to astound and amaze your friends, to give a psychological lift (if no other!) and to say, "I'm being good to me, taking the time to give myself something very specially delicious and soothing and nice." They are *not* magic potions (no matter what "special secret" ingredient they boast). So enjoy them, take them for what they are, and discount all the flapdoodle that surrounds them: all the eye-of-newt-and-toe-of-frog-fountain-of-youth nonsense, all the claims and veiled promises and hints of miracles!

What masks *can* do is stimulate your skin, give it a purely temporary but very pretty tightening and glow. Treat it to some extra special nourishment or emollient oils, cleanse it by coaxing out impurities from the pores, and pamper, pamper, pamper.

Discount mysterious muds and special mineral waters from secret, sulfurous hot springs. Try, if you like, honey or vegetable juices (at best a source of vitamins, of which only A and D penetrate the skin in sufficient amounts to be at all beneficial). Lift your face temporarily with white of egg, which tightens as it dries, feels great, then drops your chins again promptly when you smile or wash it off. (It's drying, so keep away from eye area. Also some few people—and you probably know by now if you are one— are sensitive to eggs, so if you're egg allergic, don't try it.) Keep away from powerful skin stimulants—known in the cosmetic trade as "rubefacients" (meaning "making red"). These work like mustard plasters, irritating the skin to excite a flow of blood just below the skin surface; this makes the skin look glow-y and red, and is *supposed* to cleanse the pores or the blood or something. Our cosmetic chemist says reject *all* strong rubefacients, but if you approach it in the proper frivolous spirit and you want a little drama with your t.l.c., try the masks below. Easy, fun, delicious!

Cucumber cosmetics seem to have a shorter life than most. Therefore, make 'em fresh, use 'em fresh, refrigerate 'em quick, and don't grieve if they don't last too long. *All* egg white masks are infinitely adjustable. Find the amount of egg white *you* like, to give the tightening *you* relish. Our amounts are *suggested,* not prescribed.

MILD CUCUMBER MASK

> whites of 2 eggs (about ¼ cup)
> ¼ cup plus 2 tbsp. cucumber juice
>   (one large cuke should do it)
> 2 tbsp. 90 proof vodka
> 1 tsp. lemon juice

Wash your cuke and grind it in the blender, skin and all, for more vitamins and cucumber fragrance. (If no blender, grate it carefully, catching all the juice, or put it through the finest blade of your meat chopper.) Strain the juice through triple cheesecloth, or through a nice, clean old nylon stocking. Reserve the juice, and throw away the pulp (or eat; great with salt and pepper!). You should have at least the necessary one-fourth cup plus two tablespoons. If not, start grinding another cuke.

When you have the correct amount of cucumber juice, separate your eggs and measure the egg white into a small bowl, then add the cuke juice and mix with your electric beater until smooth. Then *very* slowly add the vodka, beating constantly. At the very last, add the lemon juice, and—*voila!* MILD CUCUMBER MASK, or Vodka Sour! Makes three-fourths cup.

Cosmetic chemists are a questioning, curious bunch, and if you're getting to be one at all, you should be asking right this moment, "Why vodka?" Well—vodka is defined by U.S. law as just water and alcohol, period; no flavor added. Ninety proof means 45 percent alcohol plus water, unadulterated, therefore nice and pure for your cosmetics. There's no odor to speak of, and it's *different*, and besides, Dr. T. *loves* Vodka Sours.

(If you don't, about four teaspoons of 70 percent *ethanol* rubbing alcohol will give more or less the same results. But *don't* try to drink it!)

STRONG CUKE MASK

> whites of 3 eggs (about ¼ cup plus 2 tbsp.)
> ¼ cup cucumber juice (one large cuke should be more than enough)
> 2 tsp. lemon juice
> 2 tbsp. vodka
> 40 drops (about ¼ tsp.) peppermint extract

Wash, grind and strain cuke as for MILD CUCUMBER MASK, above.

Mix your egg whites (why not use the yolks for LECITHIN BASE; *see* Base Stocks) and cuke juice, beating with electric beater until smooth.

Then *very* slowly add vodka, lemon juice, and peppermint extract, beating constantly. Behold—a smooth, mint-green, heavenly-smelling, kick-y, lift-y mask. Makes a bit less than a cup.

For a clingier mask, add one tablespoon honey, if it pleases you. Or, as with all egg white masks, vary the amount of egg white to get exactly the tightening effect you like best. If your teen-age daughter wants to have a go at it (or your teen-age son; boys get pimples, too!), try whipping in one-fourth *cake* of USP grade camphor (*not* mothballs; *not* the same at all!). You can buy one-half and one-ounce cakes in your drugstore; one-fourth cake is about one-eighth of an ounce. Crumble it up, whip it in, and take advantage of the *azulene* in the camphor, which should help dry up the teen-age uglies.

PEPPERMINT MASK
(for a *cold* HOT lift)

white of egg (about 2 tbsp.)
1 tsp. dry gum tragacanth
½ cup water
¼ tsp. pure peppermint extract
1–2 drops green food color

Measure out all ingredients into a small bowl, beat together with electric mixer until thoroughly mixed, smear on face, and say *wow!*

At first it feels cool, thanks to the peppermint oil (a source of *menthol*); then, because you've put a whopping good dose of menthol in—as we told you to—it begins to feel *warm*. (A *pink*efacient?) Finally, about five minutes after application, it glosses over and you feel a bit of tightening, and the show is over.

Leave it on, take it off, makes not a bit of difference. It won't hurt you, like some of those Hungarian goulashes that are so active they have to be removed prompto—or else. This one can be washed off with clear, cool water, leaving a nice bright glow behind. If you want just the *cool* part of the mask, cut the peppermint in half. ("Note:" says Dr. T., "hot and cold running masks our specialty.")

In this and in other recipes calling for gum trag, gum arabic can be substituted. Gum arabic in lump form can be rolled with a rolling pin in a plastic bag for easier powdering. It dissolves more rapidly in a heated water solution but be sure to cool before mixing with egg white!

CHAPTER EIGHT

TREATMENTS

LUXURY THROAT STICK

¼ cup plus 1 tbsp. sesame oil
1 tbsp. beeswax
2 tbsp. paraffin wax
2 tbsp. cocoa butter

Measure all the ingredients into a small enamel saucepan (see Tricks of the Trade for hints on melting beeswax and paraffin) and warm slowly over hot water, either in double boiler or electric fry pan. Stir together thoroughly.

When completely melted, pour into a jar (in which case you have to apply it with your fingers), or into an old plastic stick deodorant container which you or your husband may have around. If you use this, clean it out thoroughly first, and *push the base all the way down until it touches bottom*. Then pour in your molten mixture and let stand undisturbed until it hardens completely. If you're anxious, put it into the refrigerator for a few hours to speed the process up. Then push up the stick and—wow! a lovely, unctuous, almost-white stick of just the right consistency to smooth onto your throat. (Rub *up;* the slight friction gives a stimulating, massaging effect which is good for you, too.)

The stick liquefies on contact and you feel the difference immediately! If you like you can add a drop or two of food coloring and a bit of perfume *after* you take your mixture off the hot water and *before* it reaches the hardening stage, but we like this stick just as it is, creamy white with a rich smell of cocoa butter. It's great for wrinkles, too, for dry hands that need a touch of luxury treatment, and, *my* mama used to say, for the front of ladies' fronts, to keep the skin there smooth and elastic and right where it's supposed to be! Makes about one-half cup.

Glidey LUXURY THROAT STICK is a beauty, one of the small triumphs our cosmetic chemist preened himself over almost unbearably. A simpler version, not so luxurious but also meltingly rich and smelling sweetly of cocoa butter is VICTORY THROAT STICK, a good bet if you can't find the slightly exotic sesame oil and beeswax called for, for true LUXURY.

If you want to be kind to VICTORY THROAT STICK and yourself, dress it up by adding a bit of safflower oil, or even real butter, for richness (and vitamins!). The formula is deliberately a little stiff so that you can play around with it in this fashion.

VICTORY THROAT STICK

> 2 tbsp. paraffin
> 3 tbsp. cocoa butter
> 2 tbsp. hydrogenated (solid) vegetable shortening
> *If desired:* 1 to 2 tsp. safflower oil, butter, or . . . what have you?

Melt all ingredients together over water, as in LUXURY THROAT STICK, mix well, pour either into jar or into empty, cleaned out, *pushed down* stick deodorant case. Cool. Makes a scant half cup.

By now you should have noticed that in both LUXURY and VICTORY THROAT STICKS, cocoa butter is a major ingredient. "What's so special about cocoa butter?" well you may ask. For one thing, it's gorgeously rich in polyunsaturates, which means that it's right at home with normal skin oils and can sneak down into pores to do deep lubrication where it counts. For another, cocoa butter has a low melting temperature, just above normal body heat, a lovely plus because it stays creamy in your formula, but the slight friction involved in applying it to your skin liquefies it immediately—ergo: no greasy, waxy feel, and, superemolliency. Cocoa butter was and is used in luxury cosmetics, but most manufacturers find it too expensive for less costly lines. There's also a problem of perishability which you, dear home cosmetic chemist, with your refrigerator and your realistic outlook about fresh ingredients (*see* A Note About Preservatives) don't need to worry your head about. So all in all, cocoa butter is an elegant, natural, time-tested cosmetic ingredient which manufacturers are seldom able to give you (and when they do, they *boast* about it in big letters, thank you!) but you, at home, can, and will, make handsome use of.

BEAUTY SCRUB

Active Base:
   ¼ tsp. camphor USP (*not* mothballs or flakes!)
   2 tbsp. 70% *ethanol* rubbing alcohol
   2 tbsp. 70% isopropyl rubbing alcohol
   2 tbsp. clear liquid shampoo
   1 tsp. lemon juice

The Grains:
   ¾ cup *old fashioned* oatmeal (*not* instant
      or 5 minute!)

(To get your one-fourth teaspoon camphor USP, buy a half-ounce cake at your drug store, crumble it, and measure out one-fourth teaspoon.)

Dissolve the camphor in the two alcohols. (A good way is to shake them up together in a small bottle, so that the alcohol doesn't evaporate.) Then add the liquid shampoo and the lemon juice, and stir (or shake) until clear. If necessary, warm the mixture slightly by holding a *capped* bottleful under very hot running water. *Don't* boil up, either directly or over boiling water.

You now have an active drying base, which can be used by itself on extra-oily teen-age skin, or, much more elegantly, combined with oatmeal to make a brisk, cooling BEAUTY SCRUB, as follows:

Work Active Base into oatmeal, about two tablespoons at a time, crumbling between your fingers until thoroughly absorbed. Work fast, so that the alcohol won't evaporate. The grittier the oatmeal you see, the more abrasive your Beauty Grains will be, and conversely—if your skin is too sensitive to like much stimulation, the quicker-cooking the oatmeal, the softer and mushier the scrub.

When the scrub is thoroughly mixed, put it in a wide mouth jar, and cap tightly. To use: just wet your face, use one-half to one teaspoon of scrub, and lather up a storm. As with *all* alcohol products, keep away from eyes.

If after you've used it awhile, the scrub seems to lose its zip, simply work in a bit more Active Base. If, on the other hand, it's too zippy for your comfort, make it up with only *ethanol* alcohol next time. (For more zip, increase the proportion of *isopropyl*.)

If your teen-ager has real problem skin, try dissolving a pinch of salicylic acid (a mild antiseptic you can buy at your drug store) in the Active Base before working it into the grains. Pimples, avast! Try it.

CUCUMBER SKIN TONER

First phase:
    1 whole egg
    ¼ cup peanut oil
    ½ cup plain yogurt

Second phase:
    2 tbsp. SUSPENSION JELLY (*See* Base Stocks)
    2 tbsp. lemon juice
    ¼ cup plus 1 tbsp. witch hazel
    1 whole cucumber

Beat the egg until white and yolk are thoroughly mixed. Add peanut oil and beat again until egg disperses smoothly. Then add yogurt, and beat with electric mixer on *high* to get a smooth lotion.

Now stir together the SUSPENSION JELLY, the lemon juice, and the witch hazel until there are no lumps at all. Wash the cucumber and grind it whole, skin and all, in a meat grinder or blender, or grate it, *losing none of the juice*. Put pulp and juice through fine cheesecloth to strain; let the liquid settle, and pour off the clear top layer to use. (Eat the rest of the cucumber if you want to; it's delicious with salt and pepper!)

Add one-fourth cup clear cucumber juice to the other ingredients in the *second phase*.

Now slowly add the juice portion (second phase) to the cream portion (first phase), beating constantly with electric mixer on *slow* speed. When everything's in, and *thin,* beat for a few more moments at slow speed, then bottle. Or better still, slap it right on your face and feel the cool, heavenly cucumber feel, smell the fresh green smell, and enjoy the slight tingly tightening feeling of the egg white plus the protein nourishment of the yolk. Makes about two cups.

FRESH CUCUMBER SKIN TONER is more perishable than most of the cosmetics you'll make (not much preservative in it—only the bit of witch hazel), so you may want to add twelve drops of merthiolate to help keep it fresh. In any case, your label should read:

Keep Refrigerated. Shake Before Using.

POUSSE CAFE "MAGIC" LOTION

Oil phase:
    1 tbsp. lanolin
    1 tbsp. cocoa butter
    ⅓ cup light mineral oil
    3 tbsp. peanut oil
    1 tsp. almond extract or your perfume choice

Water phase:
   2 tbsp. water
   1 tbsp. glycerine
   ¼ cup plus 2 tbsp. 70% *ethanol* rubbing alcohol
   1 drop blue food coloring (or your color choice)

First the oil phase:

In a small enamel saucepan, measure out all the oil phase ingredients except the almond extract, and heat them slowly over hot water (as detailed in Tricks of the Trade) until completely melted together. Remove from water and allow to cool. While cooling, add the almond extract, or one teaspoon of another food flavor, or one teaspoon of your favorite fragrant bath oil. (Use only *floating* bath oil here, not the type that disperses in a milky lotion when added to water.) If you're really extravagant, you can try about ten drops of your favorite perfume. In any case:

Now the water phase:

Combine the water, glycerine and alcohol and stir together until completely dissolved. (You may, at this point, choose to substitute your favorite splash cologne—perhaps the one you made—for all or part of the alcohol. Do *not* use *isopropyl* alcohol, though, as it has a harsh odor and tends to sting a bit. If you *do* use a splash cologne, you can leave out the perfume or food flavor extract in the oil phase.) Add a drop of food color to the mixture now—*not* yellow, though.

The mix:

Combine the water and oil phases in a large bottle— twelve ounces will do nicely—and shake vigorously, then quickly pour out into smaller bottles if desired. A little bit of this rich formula will go a long way, and you may enjoy giving some away as striking gifts. Because not only is POUSSE CAFE an excellent treatment for normal or dry skin, it's also absolutely beautiful. As the lotion stands, it separates into three layers: the golden oil phase on top, the clear blue (or your favorite color) water phase on the bottom, and a "mixed" layer (aqua, if blue was your color) in the middle. Shake the bottle and it recombines into a striking opaque aqua (or orange or . . .) lotion, then separates out again in about half an hour. A truly magic potion!

POUSSE CAFE is especially enriching as a throat lotion. The combination of lanolin and cocoa butter with the oils leaves a velvety skin feel which is an excellent protective veil against wind and sun and wonderful for dry, "crepey" skin. The glycerine gives "humectancy"—that is, it helps hold moisture to the skin. The alcohol content cuts the oily feel as you apply the lotion, yet it soon evaporates on the skin. It is *not* drying in this context. Witch hazel could be substituted for part or all of the alcohol in POUSSE CAFE, but it doesn't give quite as dramatic effects in the color separation.

Concocting POUSSE CAFE is a valuable lesson in cosmetic chemistry, too. Most of the creams and lotions you use— and will make—are *emulsions,* mixtures of water and oil in which the droplets of one are permanently suspended (enrobed) in droplets of the other. Mayonnaise is an emulsion; so is milk (butterfat droplets suspended in water). Most permanent emulsions are kept stable by the presence of an emulsifier, a substance which breaks down the natural resistance between water and oil droplets, and encourages them to mix. Sometimes emulsions are stabilized merely by superpowerful mixing or beating, e.g., the homogenization of milk. But we'll use emulsifiers, mostly natural ones like lanolin or egg yolk.

POUSSE CAFE is that rare creature, a temporary emulsion. Shake it and you can see the emulsion form, hold for awhile, then gradually separate back into its transparent water and oil components. The color trick is based on the fact that the food coloring dissolves in the water but not in the oil. As the water and oil layers separate, all the dye is seen where it belongs—in the water. Only while there is an emulsion is there a mixture of colored water and yellow oil.

"Why do we want an emulsion at all?" we asked Dr. T. Because merely smearing oil or grease on our faces is an unpleasant sensation, unaesthetic, unbeautiful. Oil droplets robed in water feel pleasant on the skin, cool and velvety rather than greasy, and much less oil is needed to get the maximum emollient benefits.

So *make* POUSSE CAFE, *shake* POUSSE CAFE, and *take* POUSSE CAFE—to all of your friends; a dramatic, personal, and luxurious skin liqueur.

Label: Shake Before Using.

(Just for fun, Dr. Tibor tried chocolate in the POUSSE CAFE as a substitute for cocoa butter. "Same properties, felt fine, but looked awful," he reports. "I tossed it out promptly.")

HANDY HUBBY BODY RUB

¼ cup lanolin
¼ cup sesame oil (or safflower, if it's easier for you to find)
3 tbsp. oil of wintergreen (methyl salicylate)
½ cup plus 1 tbsp. water

Measure lanolin, sesame oil, and oil of wintergreen into a medium-size enamel pan and heat it slowly over hot water until thoroughly melted together. Stir, then remove from hot water and allow to cool. When it's at room temperature, slowly add the water, beating constantly with electric mixer on *high*. Beat for a few seconds after all water is added, to make sure you have a smooth, even emulsion.

This makes about one and one-fourth cups of rich, body-rubbing lotion of the type athletes (and home handymen!) use to work out sore, stiff, or sprained muscles. Rub it on briskly and it develops heat where applied; it feels great, smells strong, goes on pleasantly, and is an even, stable emulsion. It's not as strong as some commercial preparations of this type, which use menthol, camphor, etc. to irritate the skin mildly; the body then rushes blood to this part of the skin which produces the hot effect strong men love. But HANDY HUBBY works up sufficient heat when applied to give a soothing effect, and leaves an absolutely elegant, velvety feel on the skin. Great after a long, hard day of plastering ceilings!

As with all oil of wintergreen products, HANDY HUBBY should be labelled:

Do Not Swallow. Keep Away From Children.

CHAPTER NINE

A GENERAL NOTE ON BATH PRODUCTS

Bathing has come a long way since the days when, if you were lucky, you thoroughly immersed yourself *maybe* once a week, in an iron tub into which somebody poured boiling water heated on a coal stove. You cleansed yourself with rough homemade cakes of soap, and then only because you couldn't *stand* yourself otherwise—and all the while *some* folks hinted darkly that bathing could kill you, or at the very least weaken your muscles and make your hair fall out.

Today, bathing is an art! Cosmetic counters are full of bath oils, bath salts, bubble baths, bath powders, floating, bubbling, dispersing and nondispersing—not to mention *after* bath products, splashes and frictions and colognes. What's the difference between them? Sometimes there's very little. In one way or another, in varying degrees, they all try to do what bath oil was originally designed for—to smooth and condition your skin after bathing, make it feel good, smell good, make bath time a special, luxurious occasion.

Bath oils come in two forms: *floating* oils and *dispersing* oils. Both usually look pretty much the same: clear, pretty liquids. But try the eyedropper test on them and you'll see the difference. Carefully place a few drops of each on the surface of its own glass of clean warm water. The floating oil, if properly formulated, will seem to explode as it hits the water, instantly forming a very thin film on *top*. The dispersing oil will explode, too, but what a difference! It will swirl *through* the water, dispersing oil *evenly throughout*. The floating oil is the one manufacturers love best; it needn't be as rich or as generously perfumed as the dispersing oil, since it's all concentrated on top, instead of spread out and diluted in twenty gallons or so of water. But it's the *dispersing* oil *you* should be after, just because it's rich and well perfumed, *and* coats you from head to toe in an emollient treatment for as long as you soak blissfully in your tub. GOLDEN GLOVE, EGG-CREAM BATH OIL is this kind of product, as you'll soon discover. Read on!

After bath splash is essentially a cologne with some alcohol-soluble oil in it to counteract the drying effect of the cologne and provide an emollient film after bathing. You're making virtually the same thing when you concoct an after shave. (See after shave recipes for more details.)

"Bubbling bath oil" is often a poor quality bubble bath to which oil has been added, thereby cutting down the foaming power. Bath powders are generally just talc plus a good fragrance plus (usually) some sort of fat worked into it to reduce the drying property of straight talc. Perfume bath oils are just perfume oil cut with another very light oil (usually a material called a "fatty acid ester") instead of alcohol. Alcohol is almost always used in perfumes, colognes, and toilet waters, because it evaporates quickly and gives a lift to the fragrance. But perfume bath oils—and all fragrant bath oil products—count on the heat of your tub water to do the lifting for them. The newest and most dazzling of the after bath cosmetics, the veil, is a more complicated cologne emulsion, containing 30 to 50 percent alcohol to give lift to even the most delicate fragrances, yet also containing various emollient esters and oils. The whole thing is held together by a type of gum which is not available to the home cosmeticook.

But, hosanna, your EGG-CREAM BATH OIL is as good as any of them. Hurray for Dr. T.!

EGG-CREAM BATH OIL (GOLDEN GLOVE)

1 whole egg
½ cup sesame oil (or substitute safflower oil)
1 tsp. liquid dishwashing detergent
2 tbsp. 70% *isopropyl* rubbing alcohol
¼ cup milk
¼ tsp. orange or lemon extract or perfume of
    your choice

Beat the egg and the sesame oil together until smooth, using *medium* speed of your electric mixer. Then *slowly* add the detergent while you continue beating. A smooth pale gold lotion will form at this point.

Now *very slowly* add the alcohol (which will thin the mixture again), and then the milk. The milk will be a bit difficult to work in, but keep beating.

Now work in the perfume—orange or lemon extract is scrumptious, or, if you want something really exotic, use your favorite cologne or friction lotion in place of part or all of the alcohol. Another trick to get your favorite fragrance is to substitute some of your favorite scented bath oil for part of the sesame oil. Makes one cup.

GOLDEN GLOVE, says Dr. T. proudly, is different from any bath oil you've ever used. It's a rich emulsion, which sets up after a few hours, either to a thick lotion or to a light cream, depending on what substitutions you may have made. Better use a wide-necked bottle, as it may not want to pour out of a narrow one. If this should happen, though, don't panic; simply recap your bottle, hold it under hot running water, and GOLDEN GLOVE will thin dutifully and flow. Handle this product with love and appreciation; you've obviously got a richer, more emollient, more skin-loving-and-nourishing a product here than any commercial formulator could afford to make, or could keep fresh enough to sell.

What's more, GOLDEN GLOVE is a true dispersing bath oil, not the floating, greasy, ring-around-the-tub variety. Want to prove it? Zoop up a few drops in any eyedropper.

(What? You haven't got one yet? Shame! Run right out and buy one! It's absolutely essential for all sorts of cosmeticookery, from adding drops of coloring solution to drops of perfume or flavor extracts, to tests such as this.) Drop two or three drops of your newly made GOLDEN GLOVE onto the surface of a glass of very clean warm water, and watch the drops explode as they spread over the water. Now give a twirl with your fingers or a spoon and you'll see the whole glass become milky. (If yours doesn't do this, you've done something wrong!)

If you want to see the dramatic difference, make the same test with whatever bath oil *you've* been using. Chances are it will bead and float on the surface, leaving the rest of the water clear.

Why is a dispersing bath oil so extra specially desirable? A floating bath oil which hugs the surface and leaves the rest of the water clear doesn't do you a particle of good while you soak; it merely gives you a quick "coating" of oil in the moment it takes for you to whisk up out of the water and climb over the side of the tub. It's main accomplishment is to coat the sides of your tub with a film of oil as the water goes down, leaving a sticky mess for unoiled you to scrub away. A dispersing bath oil, on the other hand, silkens you with emollients *all* the time you are in the bath water and is, moreover, somewhat kinder to the sides of your tub. It doesn't feel greasy at all, yet it soothes and gently lubricates the itchy dry-skin scales that almost everybody suffers from some time or other—especially in fall, when that sunburn starts to fade, or in winter, when indoor heat dries out your body skin. For old folks, dry-skin itch generally is a year-round complaint; try giving your parents, or your in-laws, a (wide-mouthed!) bottle of GOLDEN GLOVE, and watch them fall all over themselves praising it—and you.

The egg yolk in G.G. provides the protein for nourishing and conditioning the skin. The egg white (albumin), helps hold your emulsion together when you add the alcohol, which is needed to provide the spreading quality, but normally breaks emulsions (causes them to separate). And don't worry about the alcohol in G.G. *drying* your skin.

The tiny bit present in a tablespoon of G.G.—which is all you'll need for each tubful (maybe twenty gallons!) of bath water—will evaporate after doing its bit to help G.G. spread and disperse properly. The detergent is included in G.G. as an added emulsifier; it helps the oil and water phases (actually milk and alcohol) to hold together, thus keeping the product stable. The milk is added protein for the skin. It isn't absolutely necessary, but it adds a touch of luxury—the difference between a very good product and a great one!

The biggest problem area is the alcohol (or cologne substitution). If you should leave it out, the product would tend to glob up on the surface of the bath water, meaning you'd have to swoosh it around with your hand to disperse the oil. If you should use too much, your product will separate in the bottle within a few hours, which is no *real* problem (if you've just committed an ounce or two of precious cologne, don't weep!). You'll just have to remember to shake before using.

CHAPTER TEN

HAIR, HAIR!

In any measurable terms—weight or size or function—hair is an inconsiderable part of the human body. Yet in hours and dollars spent fussing and coaxing it, cutting and growing it, washing and brushing and combing and curling and dyeing and drying and conditioning it—hair probably takes first prize. Look at the cosmetics counters in your drugstore. Lo! hair products lead all the rest. Hair grooms, hair conditioners, hair dyes, shampoos, creme rinses, hair sprays, hair sets—we couldn't begin to name all of the bewildering variety of products that are manufactured. And yet, assuming that you have no *serious* problems with your hair (and with the exception of hair sprays and hair dyes, which are obviously out of kitchen range!) you can probably cook up at home all the basic hair products you and your family crave.

The papa of the house probably uses a hair groom, and maybe the mama or some of the kids do, too. Why? What does it do? What is it *supposed* to do?

First off, a hair groom should make the hair *manageable*—easy to comb and willing to stay in place. It must give sheen (life) to the hair, especially in this day and age when synthetic shampoos and gummy hair sprays and powerful hair dyes and bleaches combine to make the hair lifeless-looking, dull, and strawlike. But though you want your sheen, you also demand of your hair groom that it *not* be heavy and oiling; you want grooming ability *without* a plastered-down look, comb-ability *without* limpness, and so on and so on. That's why it's not enough just to smear on any old handy oil or bear grease (even though they've all been advocated and used over the centuries for hair-taming: butter, cocoa butter, mineral oil, heavy greases, tallow, fats, sperm oil, vegetable oils, mink and turtle and what-have-you oils!).

The hair grooms Dr. T. offers fulfill *all* the basic requirements we listed, and then some. They're suitable for men, women, or children; they're made from odorless oils so you can perfume them to your heart's content, *and* they're compounded from readily available materials.

Besides hair grooms, your family, or some member of it (probably you!) will long for a hair *conditioner,* a rich nutrient lotion that helps counteract the depredations of sun, salt water, drying soaps, dyes, teasing. Dr. T. has concocted several beauties, including one superior one especially for damaged hair.

Your husband, or your son (or you) may be partial to brilliantine (from the French word *briller,* to shine). Men generally prefer the solid variety, women the liquid. Solid brilliantines are (slightly) more complicated than the liquid variety. They're basically petrolatum (petroleum jelly, and for heaven's sake, get the white kind, not that sticky, ooky, awful yellow variety!) which is sometimes cut with mineral oil to soften them, sometimes stiffened with mineral wax, then perfumed to your taste. A word of caution, though: not every perfume dissolves in mineral oil (and food color *won't*). So before you commit your precious, beloved fragrance to the experiment, try a drop or two first, to make sure it'll mix.

An offshoot of brilliantine that's become *very* popular, selling in the millions of bottles per year, is a conditioner that's really only brilliantine plus lanolin. Dr. T. includes a recipe for this type of conditioning brilliantine, as well as one for the classic brilliantine, and a special stiff one for crew haircut devotees.

A mighty seller in the hair products market is shampoo, which is a second cousin to bubble bath; the main difference is that bubble bath only has to bubble, while shampoo has to *condition* as well. Notice we don't say "clean" the hair. It's a well-known fact in the cosmetic trade that the shampoos which clean the best sell the least, and vice versa. What milady wants is *not* really good cleaning, although she says she does, because when the hair is really clean, it's flyaway—it doesn't stay in place. Static electricity builds up in it just from the air friction caused by walking here and there. What's needed is a light coating which is electrically conductive, so that this static electricity can bleed off—the kind of coating that's provided by a creme rinse, or, to some extent, by any film of oil, such as that left on your hair by the indifferently cleansing (but dramatically foaming!) shampoo you are probably using now. If your current shampoo does a *good* job of cleansing, you're almost certainly using a creme rinse afterwards—which adds sheen and conditioners, de-statics, but leaves your hair limp as an undertaker's handshake. What to do, what to do?

Our mamas called a good shampoo one which would lather even in the hardest water and not form a scum on the hair due to it. Nowadays all shampoos on the market can do this; the difference lies in the amount and quality of the conditioners used. The happy medium is a shampoo that cleans *most dirt* off the hair but doesn't remove too much of the natural oils (or replaces them by having oil as an ingredient) and supplies conditioners, which are mildly substantive to the hair, that is, stick to it even in the presence of the basic soap or detergent that's supposed to remove foreign matter.

Dr. T. satisfies these requirements by starting with the cheapest clear supermarket shampoo you can find (the one he tested out cost only sixty-nine cents per quart!) and adding superluxuriant conditioners, principally whole egg, which gives protein to body the hair. A tiny bit of light oil could also be added to the recipes, though it would tend to cut the amount of foam (just psychological anyway—foam doesn't *clean,* it just foams), and beer can be used, too, if you don't mind the heady (oops!) aroma.

Any of the shampoo recipes (or your supermarket shampoo) can be gelled merely by adding one tablespoon of unflavored gelatin powder per cup and beating with your electric mixer until thoroughly dissolved (about 2 minutes). It will set up overnight, and is a nice trick—plus practical if you have kids who shampoo their own hair and tend (as mine do) to pour *all* the liquid out of the bottle every time.

Incidentally, you're also adding conditioning to your shampoo by thickening it this way, since gelatin is also a protein and quite substantive to the hair—therefore an excellent conditioner.

As for wave sets, most of the commercial sets and sprays are based on *synthetic* gums which simply aren't available to the home cosmeticook. Natural gums work quite well, though, and Dr. T. shows you how. If you chance on a supply of *karaya* (a natural gum you sometimes encounter in art supply stores or botanical houses) try it in this context, in about the same proportion as the gum tragacanth mentioned in the recipes. Another ingredient that works, and can be substituted, is plain old pectin, which you buy at your supermarket for thickening homemade jams and jellies. And see Dr. T.'s amazing revelations about citrate of magnesia, a product *we* remember as a child with something less than ecstasy. As a wave set ingredient, though, it's really something special!

PESKY CURL WAVE SET

> 2 tbsp. citrate of magnesia
> 1 cup of water
> few drops rose soluble perfume oil
> drop food color (blue is our choice)

Simply mix all ingredients together, set your hair (as with any water set) and stand back! You'll be delighted with the results—good body and elegant sheen, excellent holding power, no tackiness or gumminess. Again, you can increase the strength by stepping up the citrate of magnesia slightly and cutting back on the water.

Yes, you're right, citrate of magnesia *is* what you're thinking; you buy it in drugstores for quite another purpose. But during the thirties, flappers used it to fasten down those patent-leather shingle bobs, and it's still great, cut 'way back with water, for today's hairdos. Used straight, it will tame pesky curls, guiches, or cowlicks instanter.

WAVE SET

1 tsp. gum tragacanth powder
¾ cup water
¼ cup 70% *ethanol* rubbing alcohol
drop or two food coloring
3 drops glycerine
few drops perfume

Sprinkle gum tragacanth on the surface of the water and stir thoroughly. *Keep it moving,* so it won't form an angry, sticky lump. (If it does, you can heat the solution, which will dissolve it, but with care you won't have to.) Then add the glycerine, alcohol, food color, and perfume, and stir thoroughly. Let the mixture set overnight to thicken, bottle it, and it's ready for use.

Too much glycerine will make your WAVE SET tacky. Too much gum trag, or too little glycerine, may make your setting unpleasantly stiff. So vary the proportions to suit yourself. The alcohol will evaporate and hasten drying, so you can get out on that date faster.

A thick solution can be dipped up with the fingers; a thin one can be sprayed with an atomizer (or an old glass-cleaner bottle with a spray head). So have fun with this one; it's simple, and *very* effective.

EASY EGG SHAMPOO

1 whole egg
1 cup any brand clear (cheap) shampoo

Beat egg until smooth. Then, while *beating* (use *slow* speed or you'll be overwhelmed with foam) add the egg to the cup of shampoo. The result is a translucent shampoo which will usually clear on standing. It will have *more foam* than the original, and give beautiful conditioning. It's short-lived, though, because of the fresh egg, so refrigerate, and use up within a week or two.

SUPER-PROTEIN EASY EGG SHAMPOO

1 recipe EASY EGG SHAMPOO
or
1 whole egg
1 cup any brand clear (cheap) shampoo

and

1 packet (1 tbsp.) clear unflavored gelatin

Make EASY EGG SHAMPOO by beating the egg, then *slowly while beating,* adding it to the clear shampoo.

Then beat in *slowly* one packet of gelatin, sprinkling it on the surface of the mixture to avoid ugly lumps. Beat two minutes at the slowest speed of your electric beater. The mixture will thicken somewhat immediately, and will *gel* if you heat it up for about ten minutes *slowly* in a double boiler, or over hot water (*not* over direct heat, ever, or it'll foam over and you'll have a horrible mess!). This shampoo has double conditioning and is really fantastic for damaged, dry, or bleached hair. You can, of course, gel any shampoo merely by adding the gelatin and leaving out the egg, but the double-double effect of both is something you'll tell your friends about! Gelatin is a superior conditioner and, as you know if you've ever had broken-fingernail troubles, an excellent source of protein.

SUPER-PROTEIN EASY EGG SHAMPOO also makes a glorious SUPER-PROTEIN EASY BUBBLE BATH. Try it and see! You might want to treat yourself to a little more perfume for the bubble bath—a bit of rose geranium oil is lovely—and perhaps a drop of red food color to give you a really rosy outlook. Yummy.

GLOSSY HAIR GROOM

⅓ cup light mineral oil
2 tsp. castor oil
2½ tsp. lanolin
½ cup sesame oil
2 to 7 drops perfume *oil*

Put all ingredients except perfume oil into a small enamel pan and warm gently over hot water until the lanolin melts. Stir.

Take pan off heat, and add the perfume oil. This can be one drop rose geranium oil (strong but very spicy and intriguing: try your druggist), or a few drops of rum flavoring (supermarket) or a creation of your own—but it *must* be oil-soluble, since this recipe contains neither water nor alcohol.

Bottle GLOSSY HAIR GROOM in a handsome bottle with a small opening. Use only a few drops at a time; spread on fingers and work into hair. Makes one cup.

GLOSSY HAIR GROOM may get slightly hazy when it cools. Don't worry; it's just the lanolin and doesn't affect the product at all.

CREAM OIL HAIR GROOM

1 recipe GLOSSY HAIR GROOM
or
⅓ cup light mineral oil
2 tsp. castor oil
2½ tsp. lanolin
½ cup sesame oil
2–7 drops perfume oil

and

2 tbsp. 70% *ethanol alcohol*

Warm gently until melted together, as in GLOSSY HAIR GROOM, above. Take off heat, add perfume, and cool to room temperature.

Now pour the cooled mixture into a bottle of at least one and one-half cup capacity, which can be tightly capped. Add the two tablespoons *ethanol* alcohol, cap the bottle, and *shake hard*. Instantly, a lovely creamy emulsion will form. It will last about two hours, then break (start to separate and get less white as the globules of oil start to come out of the alcohol), so remember to shake before using—thus reconstituting the emulsion each time.

This cream oil recipe is quite similar to many brands now on the market which are sold almost exclusively in men's barber shops, where they are very popular. Ask your husband how many are lined up in front of the barber's mirror, and how many times he's paid an extra twenty-five to thirty-five cents for the privilege of letting the barber shake a few drops on as a finishing touch to his haircut.

Both GLOSSY and CREAM OIL HAIR GROOMS are fine for women and children, too. Don't worry, ladies, about the wee bit of alcohol in CREAM OIL drying your delicate tresses. The alcohol evaporates promptly when you apply this kind of hair groom, and leaves all the oils—the ones in the product and your own natural oils, too—behind, intact. There is actually an *advantage* to cream oil over straight oil hair grooms; the alcohol tends to *thin* the product considerably, and thus the oil is able to spread more evenly over the hair, ergo: less oil used to greater effect. It's easier to apply (just a dab will do) and you don't have to rub it over your hands first, as you do with GLOSSY.

If your hair is *very* dry, though, you'll probably be grateful for *all* the nourishing oils in GLOSSY, and prefer it over CREAM OIL every time.

You are by now (or should be!) enough of a cosmetic chemist (kitchen variety) to ask: why these ingredients? What do they contribute? Dr. T. answers.

The sesame oil (as mentioned previously you *could* substitute safflower if sesame is too hard to get, but have

you tried your health food store?) is very light-bodied and
not-too-oily in feel, thus reducing the overall oiliness of the
recipe to a pleasing level. (Safflower oil is slightly heavier.)
Also, sesame is highly *unsaturated,* and acts as a superb
conditioner both for the skin *and* the hair. It tends to
penetrate, whereas the mineral oil stays on the surface; thus
in this recipe the mineral oil provides the gloss. Finally,
lanolin adds just a touch of drag to help hold the hair in
place (which wouldn't be the case if your recipe were just
pure sheen and slipperiness). Also lanolin helps to form
an absorption base—holding moisture *from* the air *onto*
the hair—as well as being itself an excellent hair conditioner. The castor oil (don't say ugh!) is a favorite ingredient in hair products because it's what is known in the
trade as a drying oil—which means that it stiffens (eventually) into a sort of crusty gel when exposed to the air,
thus giving a bit of body to the hair when used in reasonably small quantities. If you'd like to modify GLOSSY, or
any hair groom to give more of this effect (for some men's
products, lots of this oil is used, and a familiar slight crust
which holds the hair immovable for *hours* is the result)
just add castor oil within reason, testing as you go.

BRILLIANTINE

2 tsp. paraffin
¼ cup plus 2 tbsp. petrolatum
    (*white* petroleum jelly)
1 tbsp. lanolin
2 tsp. water
drop or two of perfume *oil,*
    rose geranium, or your choice

Measure out paraffin, petrolatum, and lanolin into small
enamel pan and heat slowly over hot water until melted
together. Remove from heat. Add perfume oil, and stir.

Work the water into the mixture by beating *hard* for
about two minutes. Use highest speed of your electric
mixer.

When water is all taken up, slow-stir by hand until the BRILLIANTINE starts to cool enough to congeal. Pour into jars, and allow to cool and set up to final hardness—about the consistency of a lipstick, or solid shortening. Makes a bit more than one-half cup.

This is a stiff brilliantine, especially formulated for taming those short army-type brush cuts; send some to a boy in service. You'll like it, too, for calming wild wisps, or subduing bits of bangs or guiches that just won't stay put.

HIGH SHEEN PEARLY HAIRDRESS

> 2 tbsp. light mineral oil
> 2 tbsp. lanolin
> 2 tbsp. petrolatum (*white* petroleum jelly)
> 4 tsp. *warm* water
> drop or two perfume *oil*

Measure the oils together into a small enamel pan and melt over hot water until thoroughly mixed.

Remove from heat, and add perfume oil. Then beat in, using high speed of your electric mixer, the four teaspoons *warm* water. Continue beating until all water is absorbed and you have a lovely, creamy-white, pearly emulsion. Makes about one-half cup.

This is a very rich, high-sheen lotion, especially nourishing to dry or damaged hair.

CREME-LOTION HAIRDRESS

Oil phase:
> 2 tbsp. solid shortening
> 2 tbsp. lanolin
> 1 tbsp. petrolatum (petroleum jelly)
> 3 tbsp. castor oil

Water phase:
>   4 tsp. glycerine
>   2 tbsp. 10% SOAP STOCK
>   (*see* Base Stocks)
>   ¼ cup plus 2 tbsp. water

Perfuming:
>   ½ tsp. rum extract
>   ½ tsp. peppermint extract

Measure out the oil phase into a medium-size enamel pan or two-cup Pyrex measuring cup, making sure to scrape every bit of the fats off the spoon and into the mixture (a rubber spatula works fine). Heat over boiling water until the fats melt and the mixture is quite clear. Stir.

Meanwhile, in another small enamel pan or Pyrex measuring cup, heat the glycerine, SOAP STOCK, and water until it, also, is clear. Stir.

Turn off the source of heat under the boiling water and allow both pans to sit another five minutes, until they are very hot. Then remove them from the hot bath, and *slowly* add the water phase to the oil phase, *stirring constantly* with your electric beater at *low* speed. Continue to stir for about one minute after all the water has been added to the oil. Then set aside and let cool.

As the foam rises, scrape it off with a spoon; you don't want an aerated product. Stir occasionally by hand. (If you're impatient, you can quick cool your mixture by placing your pan in *cold* water and changing the water occasionally.) When the mixture is hand warm, it will start to thicken. Watch it carefully, and when it reaches room temperature, whip it up for about a minute, using your electric mixer on *high.* You can add the perfume at this point, using what Dr. T. recommends, or whatever perfume combination suits your fancy. (Since there's water present in this emulsion, you can use water-soluble perfumes *and* food colors, if you like.)

Now relax, and let the CREME-LOTION stand overnight. The next day, homogenize it by whipping again for about one minute at *high* speed. Jar it up, and serve it to the family. Makes about one cup of really elegant CREME-LOTION.

This is a persnickety, fussy recipe that takes time and effort, but is really worth the trouble. The product you get is equal to the best on the market, or so Dr. T. believes —and he should know! It's beautifully stable, pearly, creamy, and full of hair nourishment for the whole family. The hydrogenated vegetable oil (shortening to you) means, to a chemist, *triglycerides* galore—and these act as stabilizers for the emulsion, helping to thicken it without resorting to *waxes,* which tend to dull the hair. Lanolin adds its considerable hair-conditioning properties, plus its ability to act as an absorption base, forming water/oil emulsions when water is added. The petrolatum *plus* the lanolin give the drag so necessary for that "finished grooming" look; without it the hair would be shiny, but slide around and refuse to stay put. Castor oil helps to set the combing by forming its characteristic crust (*see* explanation under GLOSSY HAIR GROOM); also it's highly unsaturated, and therefore a good conditioner as well. The glycerine is a *humectant* (water-loving and -holding), here valuable for keeping the cream soft, so it won't form an ugly skin if you forget to cap the jar. Finally, the very tiny amount of soap acts as an auxiliary emulsifier (the lanolin is doing the main work in this department), and helps a bit, when shampoo times comes, to release the HAIRDRESS from the hair. (Don't worry about soap scum; the two tablespoons of SOAP STOCK called for is a 10 percent solution, containing one-tenth of an ounce of actual soap and nine-tenths of an ounce of water. A tenth of an ounce of soap recipe which makes over half a pound of CREME-LOTION is minuscule, yet in this instance very necessary to help stabilize the emulsion.)

A final note: CREME-LOTION HAIRDRESS *is* creamy; preparations of this consistency are usually sold in *tubes.* You may, with a little patience, be able to suck it into a clean, empty plastic shampoo tube by simply compressing the tube (creating a vacuum), and then sticking the end into the CREME-LOTION and letting go, coaxing the mixture inside. If this fails, put it in a wide mouth jar. Once it's set up, it will be hard to "dollop" out of a bottle—worse than new ketchup, and you *know* how pesky *that* is!

FIRST AID PROTEIN HAIR CONDITIONER

Oil phase:
   ¼ cup shortening
   3 tbsp. lanolin
   3 tbsp. castor oil

Water phase:
   4 tsp. glycerine
   1 tbsp. 10% SOAP STOCK
     (*see* Base Stocks)
   1¼ cups plus 2 tbsp. water

Protein–lecithin phase:
   1 whole egg
   Few drops perfume oil (your
     choice)

Measure out the oil phase into a medium-size enamel pan or two-cup Pyrex measuring cup, making sure that every bit of the fat is scraped off the spoon. Heat over boiling water until the fats melt together and the mixture is clear. Stir.

Meanwhile, heat the water phase in another small enamel pot over boiling water until it, too, is quite clear. Stir.

Turn off the heat under the boiling water and let both pans sit another five minutes, until they are very hot. Then remove from the hot bath and *slowly* add the water phase to the oil phase, *stirring constantly* with your electric mixer at *low* speed. Continue to stir for about a minute after all the water has been added. Then set aside and cool to room temperature. As foam rises, scrape it off with a spoon, to avoid an aerated product.

When the mixture is hand warm, it will start to thicken. When it's at room temperature, whip it up for about a minute with your electric mixer on *high*. Add the perfume now (water or oil soluble) but no food color, as this product has a gorgeous golden color of its own.

So far, you have made a variation of CREME-LOTION HAIRDRESS. But wait! Let your mixture stand overnight. The next day beat one fresh egg (one large or two small eggs; three tablespoons of egg is what you're after) and add the egg to your mixture, using your electric beater on *high*.

Magically your white CREME-LOTION turns into a lustrous golden conditioner, rich enough to leave a shiny satiny film when rubbed on the skin. You're not finished, though. After a few more hours, or even on the second day, the conditioner may go grainy, and should have a second whipping at high speed to homogenize it fully.

This FIRST AID is luscious on the hair, heavenly for dry flyaway tresses, and for damaged or dyed hair, a veritable godsend! You'll *feel* the difference after only one or two applications. Try it, too, for summertime hair, bleached or dried by sun, wind, or salt water. The combination of the protein and lecithin in the whole fresh egg and the rich emollients and humectants is so marvellous you'll never want to be without it!

CHAPTER ELEVEN

A WORD ABOUT EYE CREAMS

The eyes and the skin around them are among the most sensitive areas of the body; therefore the cosmetics formulated for them *must* be even more than usually pure and free from irritants. The cosmetic chemist usually keeps away from perfumes, except for the simple known-safe ones, like rose soluble, and is careful to keep eye cream formulas as basic and time-tested as possible.

The purpose of eye creams is threefold. Though nothing, repeat *nothing!,* will *cure* wrinkles, a rich lubricant with plenty of moisture-holding ingredients will soften the *appearance* of dry wrinkles by dewing and plumping up the look of the skin around and under the eyes. Secondly, a spready nonpenetrating cream or oil will cleanse the skin and remove traces of sticky black-blue-white-whatever goo eye makeup, stuff that usually is waterproof, and won't respond well to (drying) soap and water. Third, after a day of looking at all that modern eyes are forced to look at, through smog and fog and whatever else we've gucked up the air with, a nice, soothing, soft, rich-rich-a-a-h-h-h-nice-feeling cream applied around the eyes can really feel wonderfully relaxing and *go-o-o-o-d!*

Though the basic ingredients are relatively the same, eye creams, like all other creams, have evolved over the years. The more modern versions are lighter, whiter, fluffier, more elegant in texture, with a less greasy feel. Sometimes this elegance is achieved by combining the ingredients in an emulsion. (*See* Creams and Lotions.) But, curiously enough, the presence of the *water* required for an emulsion is sometimes in itself irritating to the eyes. For some people the fats and oils may be perfectly soothing and nonirritat-

75

ing, but the addition of *water,* as innocent an ingredient as can be, may cause their eyes to sting. So—to delight all tastes, our cosmetic chemist has concocted two versions of the same basic formula. The old fashioned product consists only of the oil phase. It has a lovely golden color, no perfume at all, soft texture, and easy spreadability. It's soothing and leaves a velvety skin feel. The second, more modern cream has all these virtues, plus fluffy whiteness, elegance of texture, and a soupçon of perfume. Formulate away!

GOLDEN EYE CREAM

  3 tbsp. lanolin
  4 tsp. BEESWAX BASE (2 tsp. beeswax, 2 tsp. safflower oil)
  1 tbsp. light mineral oil
  1 egg

Measure the lanolin and the mineral oil into a small enamel pan and heat over hot water until melted together. Take the pan off the hot water and let cool until the mixture almost gels.

While you're waiting, separate the egg and reserve the yolk. (Smear the white on your face if you like; it gives a lovely tightening mask-y feel and washes off with cold water.) Also, in another small enamel pan, melt together the beeswax and safflower oil of BEESWAX BASE over hot water.

When your lanolin-mineral oil mixture has almost gelled, quickly beat in (by hand, stirring with a spoon or fork) the egg yolk until it is smoothly dispersed.

Now add the molten BEESWAX BASE, and stir in thoroughly. At this point you can either pop GOLDEN EYE CREAM into a jar—it's really just goose grease but it feels wonderful!—or go on to a more elegant "modern" variation, WHIPPED EYE CREAM.

Makes a scant half cup.

WHIPPED EYE CREAM

1 recipe GOLDEN EYE CREAM
   (scant half cup)

or

   Oil phase:
     3 tbsp. lanolin
     4 tbsp. BEESWAX BASE (2 tsp. bees-
       wax, 2 tsp. safflower oil)
     1 tbsp. light mineral oil
     1 egg

and

   Water phase:
     5 drops rose soluble perfume oil
     1 tbsp. *cold* water

Combine the oil phase, melting the lanolin and mineral oil, letting cool till almost gelled, beating in the separated yolk of egg, then adding the molten BEESWAX BASE —exactly as for GOLDEN EYE CREAM.

But while mixture is still warm and fluid, add five drops of rose soluble perfume oil and then *quickly* add one tablespoon of *cold* water and whip *one full minute* at highest speed of your electric beater. Result: a lovely, satiny whipped water/oil emulsion, gloriously rich and soft and easy-spreading—almost good enough to eat!

Don't be misled by the fact that the only *apparent* difference between the two eye creams is five drops of perfume and a bit of water. They are two very different products—one a soft yellow unguent, the other a fluffy, white, much-less-oily-feeling emulsion. It is the difference between, on the one hand, egg yolks and oil, and on the other hand, mayonnaise.

The GOLDEN EYE CREAM uses lanolin for moisturizing, softening effect, and emolliency, and adds safflower oil because it's unsaturated and therefore penetrates the skin. Mineral oil helps remove traces of eye makeup and mascara left on the skin, and egg yolk provides lecithin, a natural emulsifier (as is lanolin) and a normal component of human skin fat, which gives elegance and easy spreadability.

CHAPTER TWELVE

CREAMS AND LOTIONS

So far we've made a spectrum of fairly simple cosmetic products. Now at last we've come to the aristocracy of cosmetics: creams and lotions.

The characteristic of creams and lotions is that they are *emulsions*—permanent suspensions either of oil droplets in water or of water droplets in oil.

We have already encountered a *temporary emulsion,* colorful POUSSE CAFE "MAGIC" LOTION, where the droplets of oil and water temporarily merge to form a lotion, then, after half an hour or so, separate out again. Another temporary emulsion you might be better acquainted with is vinegar and oil salad dressing. When you shake up the vinegar and oil together, they form a temporary emulsion which separates, or breaks almost immediately; *not* if you add *mustard,* however. Mustard is an *emulsion stabilizer,* which acts to keep the oil droplets dispersed in the vinegar, and if you add it to your Italian Dressing, your emulsion won't fall apart. You'll get the same *apparent result* if you add a raw egg to your dressing—but actually even more is happening. The *lecithin in the egg yolk* is an emulsifier—a substance which is partially soluble in *both* mediums and therefore acts to meld them together—and the *albumin in the egg white* is an emulsion stabilizer, acting in the same way as the mustard to hold the emulsion intact.

All emulsions consist of an *oil phase* (an oil or a combination of oily or waxy substance) and a *water phase* (water or ingredients which are soluble in water). These two phases are induced to combine, either by whipping them together, stirring them together, or simply melting them together. Like any good marriage, though, there must be witnesses; and for an emulsion to be permanent and stable there must be "witnesses," too: emulsifiers and, if needed, emulsion stabilizers.

Emulsions tend to take their character from the outside, or enrobing droplets. For instance, a water/oil emulsion (in which the water droplets are dispersed in the oil) tends to be rich-feeling and emollient, like NOURISHING CREAM. An oil/water emulsion, conversely, tends to be non-greasy, cool-feeling, and to disappear into the skin without leaving a film, like PEARLY HAND CREAM.

An emulsion is a delicate creature to make, but a beautiful, satisfying one if you manage it properly. Rather like a puff-pastry or an omelet, it demands exact timing, careful measurements, precise temperatures, and a sensitive *feel* for what's going on. If you practice getting the first three down pat, we guarantee you can develop the *feel* to the point where you can sense when an emulsion's about to come apart.

You may already have met a few *stable emulsions*— like FIRST AID PROTEIN HAIR CONDITIONER, HIGH SHEEN PEARLY HAIRDRESS, and CREME-LOTION HAIRDRESS. Now you'll meet lots more. The real heart and art of cosmeti-cookery lies in learning to master them.

WHIPPED MOISTURE CREAM

> *Oil phase:*
>   2 tsp. beeswax
>   4 tsp. lanolin
>   2 tsp. paraffin wax
>   ⅓ cup peanut oil
>   *or*
>   4 tsp. BEESWAX BASE (see Base Stocks)
>   4 tsp. lanolin
>   4 tsp. PARAFFIN WAX BASE (see Base Stocks)
>   ¼ cup peanut oil

and

Water phase:
2 tsp. glycerine
¼ tsp. borax
⅓ cup water

and

Perfume:
¼ tsp. perfume oil of your choice
1 drop food color (red, for pink,
or yellow, for gold)

Measure the oils and waxes (or Bases) into a medium-size enamel pot or two-cup Pyrex measuring cup, and heat slowly over boiling water.

Meanwhile, in another small pot, mix the glycerine, borax and water and bring to a simmer. Stir, to make sure borax is completely dissolved.

When both pots are simmering—*not boiling*—slowly add the water phase to the oil phase. Hold at a simmer for five minutes, stirring occasionally.

Now take the mixture off the source of heat and start beating slowly with hand mixer or electric mixer at *low* speed. The cream will gradually thicken and start to whiten. When it reaches the consistency of a thin mayonnaise (it will be hand warm by now) add one more tablespoon of warm water, your food color, and perfume, and continue beating.

Now you'll see a dramatic change: your mayonnaise-y mixture will suddenly whiten and thicken into an elegant, firm, glossy cream. Continue to beat as before, scraping down the sides of the bowl to avoid fatty lumps. The longer you can beat, the better your final emulsion will be, but the cream should be still slightly warm when you scoop it into jars. Don't despair, though; if you misjudge this final step, you can rewarm cream, rebeat, and try again. Makes about one cup.

Why use a moisturizer, when you can use an emollient or a nourishing cream, or both? What's so special about moisture in the skin; what does it mean, anyway? Our cosmetic chemist, Dr. T., answers by telling about a classic experiment, during the fifties, run by Dr. Irvin Blank of Harvard. Dr. Blank took samples of human callus—which is the ultimate in dry skin—and soaked them in various emollient oils. Nothing whatever happened; they weren't softened and they weren't renewed. Then he soaked the callus in plain water, and—*mirabile!* It *absorbed* the water and became soft and flexible again. From this dramatic experiment, skin experts deduced that it's not *oils* which can renew your skin, but water—*moisture.* Emollients can help feed the sebum glands in the skin and soften the appearance of dry skin lines, but *humectants,* water-loving substances which take water out of the air and *hold it* to the skin, can actually help the skin look plumped out, dewy, and softer—like the callus in Dr. Blank's test. This effect lasts *only as long* as the moisturizer is on the skin—so use WHIPPED MOISTURE CREAM generously and often, on any areas of your skin that feel dried out and scaly—and that includes elbows, heels, throat, face, area around eyes—plus, if you can bear to part with it—on *leather* bags, shoes, gloves (*not* suede, as you have no doubt figured out for yourself!).

The moisturizing agents in WHIPPED MOISTURE CREAM are lanolin—the best moisturizer, really; it's this quality that makes it so popular in cosmetics, even though it's also a superior emollient—and glycerine. Versatile lanolin wears two hats in this recipe; it's an emulsifier as well, and so is the bit of borax. The waxes give the elegant texture, and the peanut oil, emolliency.

In all, WHIPPED MOISTURE CREAM is a beautiful moisturizer that melts into the skin and is absorbed almost at once, leaves no greasy residue, and will almost certainly be one of your favorites.

If you like to experiment—and you should, home cosmeticook!—try substituting safflower or sesame oil for the peanut oil; it will give a still more penetrating and moisturizing product. To transform the basic recipe into a moisturizing cleansing cream, substitute mineral oil instead; mineral oil won't penetrate the skin at all, but will stay on the surface and help remove makeup and grease. Increasing the beeswax slightly will make a slightly stiffer cream, if that's the way you like it.

NOURISHING CREAM

Oil phase:
    ¼ cup plus 1 tsp. safflower oil
    ¼ cup plus 1 tbsp. lanolin
    ½ tsp. beeswax
    1½ tsp. paraffin wax
              or
    ¼ cup safflower oil
    ¼ cup plus 1 tbsp. lanolin
    1 tsp. BEESWAX BASE
       (*see* Base Stocks)
    1 tbsp. PARAFFIN WAX BASE
       (*see* Base Stocks)

and

Water phase:
    ¼ cup plus 1 tbsp. witch hazel
    ½ tsp. borax

and

Perfume:
    ¼ tsp. perfume oil of your choice

Optional:
    1 to 2 tsp. tincture of benzoin

Measure out all ingredients in oil phase (or alternate oil phase if you've made Base Stocks) into a medium-size enamel pot or two-cup Pyrex measuring cup and heat over boiling water until melted and clear.

Meanwhile, in a small enamel pot, heat the witch hazel to a simmer, then *remove from heat,* add the borax, and stir to dissolve. Make sure that all the grains of borax are completely gone; work them with a spatula, if necessary, to break them up. Work fast; witch hazel contains a little bit of alcohol, which adds to its astringent effect, and which can boil off if you keep it too hot for too long. Remove both pots from source of heat.

Now *slowly* add the water phase to the oil phase, stirring constantly with your electric beater on *low*. Keep beating as a beautiful, light golden-colored emulsion forms, glossy and elegant. Keep beating, working the blade of your beater around in the cream and scraping down the sides of the pan as the cream thickens. Add the perfume during this stage, and the tincture of benzoin, if you decide to use it. When the cream is quite cool, thick and glossy, spoon it into jars. If you notice any oil or water separation the next day, simply rework it (cold) and it should hold together beautifully, and indefinitely.

The term "nourishing cream" is sort of an old-fashioned one; it's really a throwback to the 1930's, when your mama or grandma used it to mean a fairly heavy cream, very rich in texture and ingredients, and quite noticeable on the skin. Later on it developed into the "night cream," which has a similar formula but is a bit lighter in texture. Traditionally, these creams were loaded with all sorts of goodies—lanolin, unsaturated oils (such as the safflower oil in our recipe), exotic extracts which somebody-or-other pronounced to be nourishing to the skin as it grew older and drier and less supple, plus, sometimes, vitamins and mildly astringent ingredients to help firm the skin.

Our recipe takes note of this tradition, and offers a truly awesome amount of lanolin, plus witch hazel, to counteract the somewhat unpleasant heavy feel the lanolin imparts. Beeswax and paraffin help create the characteristic creamy texture, and the borax helps as an emulsifier, to hold the whole creation together. You can put in or leave out the tincture of benzoin; it's mildly astringent,

but can't do too much in the presence of so much oil
phase. Still, it adds a pleasant aroma, and can act as a
mild stimulant. Dr. T. likes it here, and so do I.

Use your NOURISHING CREAM on all dry skin, heels,
throat, and elbows, as well as your face (whip up some
EYE CREAM for those nasties under and around the eyes
if you have a special problem there). It will also nourish
beloved wooden serving pieces, old leather (and for that
matter *new* leather) handbags, and (beautifully!) patent
leather shoes. Try some!

CLEANSING CREAM FOR NORMAL SKIN

Oil phase:
> ½ cup light mineral oil
> 1 tbsp. paraffin wax
> 1½ tbsp. beeswax
> > > *or*
> > > ¼ cup plus 2 tbsp. light mineral
> > > oil
> > > 2 tbsp. PARAFFIN WAX BASE (*see*
> > > Base Stocks)
> > > 3 tbsp. BEESWAX BASE (*see* Base
> > > Stocks)

and

Water phase:
> ¼ cup plus 2 tbsp. water
> *heaping* ½ tsp. measure of borax

and

Perfume:
> ¼ tsp. perfume oil of your choice

Measure the oil phase into a medium-size enamel pot
and heat it slowly over boiling water until quite hot.

Meanwhile, in a separate small enamel pot, heat the water phase, making sure the borax is totally dissolved and the solution is perfectly clear.

When the oil phase is melted together and the water phase is thoroughly dissolved, take both pots off boiling water. *Immediately,* without letting either phase cool even a bit, add water phase to oil phase, beating constantly with electric beater on *medium.*

As you continue beating, the mixture begins to cool and a beautiful white emulsion forms which thickens into a rich, lustrous cream.

Don't stop! Keep beating, slowing speed down to *low* as the cream cools further. And keep on and on, beating steadily until the cream is (don't cheat!) hand warm. Just before you finish beating, add perfume and mix in thoroughly.

You've whipped up about a cup of the most elegant, pure, effective cleansing cream you've probably ever put a finger to. It liquefies the minute you apply it to your skin, and will whisk away makeup perfectly, leaving you soft, silky, and *clean.* If you want to follow up with either ASTRINGENT or PINK PEARL SKIN FRESHENER to remove the last traces of cream, you'll have an even more velvety look and feel.

This recipe is very similar to the very first cold cream made by the Greek physician, Galen, only 100 years after the birth of Christ. Many centuries of beautiful women had known that oils would remove makeup or soil from the skin even more efficiently than water. But oils have a hot, greasy feel, and leave an unpleasant, sticky aftersensation. So Galen compounded the very first cosmetic cream ever made by patiently working water into beeswax and olive oil, a cold-feeling cream, because the wax/oil droplets were enrobed in a water base, thus creating a water/oil emulsion. Simple, yes. But for almost a thousand years, Galen's formula was compounded by generations of alchemists. And, with some small changes (notably the addition of borax as an emulsifier, which gives a more luxurious cream) you have compounded it, too!

PEARLY HAND CREAM

Oil phase:
  2 tbsp. stearic acid
  4 tsp. safflower oil

Water phase:
  2 tbsp. glycerine
  ½ tsp. clear shampoo
  ½ cup 10% SOAP STOCK (*see* Base
    Stocks)
  ¼ cup water
  2 drops red food color

Perfume:
  1 tsp. almond extract

Measure oil and stearic acid (try art or candle supply stores for this crystalline wax used in candle-making) into a medium-size pan or two-cup Pyrex measuring cup. Heat over boiling water until very hot; this may take about ten minutes.

Meanwhile measure the water phase into a small enamel pot and heat over boiling water until very hot, as with oil phase.

Remove both pots from heat, and *add water phase to oil phase in a steady stream,* beating constantly with electric beater on *high.*

When the water and oil phases are combined, *quickly* place the mixture back over boiling water, and continue to beat for three to five minutes. When you start this beating you'll have an unlovely, chunky gunk of fat and water. As you beat, however, the fats will accept the water, and the mixture will thin and smooth and become, as though by magic, a beautiful, satiny pink *lotion.* You can't beat too much at this point, so if you're not sure you have your lotion, beat on. When you *are* sure, and the change is a gradual but dramatic one, remove the pot from the boiling water, slow down your beater speed to *low,* and continue to beat (now your purpose is to *cool* the emulsion) stopping frequently to stir down the cooled, thickened cream from the sides of the pan.

When the outside of the pan is hand-warm, stir in the almond extract. As it cools, your mixture will thicken. When it's still slightly warm, but thick enough so that the beater doesn't move it much (like thick whipped cream), your HAND CREAM is finished; stop stirring and pack it into wide-mouthed jars. In a few days (thanks to the stearic acid) it will develop its elegant characteristic pearl. Makes a bit over a cup.

If you have beaten the cream too long while *cooling,* it will soften too much, lose its firm texture, and fail to develop its pearl. If that happens, don't despair. Just heat it up again to lotion consistency, and start beating and cooling again.

If you can't get hold of stearic acid, you *can* compound this cream using solid vegetable shortening for the whole oil phase, that is, one-fourth cup plus two tablespoons shortening. But you won't get as elegant a product, and it won't pearl. The secret of the stearic acid is that it crystallizes as it cools, and this crystal structure gives it a characteristic appearance and feel. When you stick your finger into a jar of cream made with stearic acid, you can feel the cream break (suddenly give and liquefy) as you rub it in. Also, stearic acid is somewhat waterproof, and thus, in this cream, it offers some protection against dishpan hands.

The safflower oil in the recipe acts to smooth out the feel of the cream; if you just used stearic acid crystals it would feel watery as you rubbed it in. Glycerine is a humectant (holds moisture in the cream as well as on the skin), and the SOAP STOCK and shampoo (any cheap clear brand will do) act as emulsifiers to hold the water and oil phases together. The red food color gives a delicious, feminine, typical hand cream color, and the almond extract is to remind you of a very famous brand of hand cream which *isn't* pink and does *not* use this formula!

LEMON CREAM

Oil phase:
   3 tbsp. lanolin
   1 tbsp. petrolatum (petroleum jelly)
   1 tbsp. mineral oil
   1 tbsp. solid vegetable shortening
                  or
   ¼ cup plus 2 tbsp. MOTHER BASE #4
      (*see* Mother Bases)

and

Water phase:
   2 tbsp. glycerine
   2 tbsp. fresh lemon juice (strained) or
      reconstituted juice
   4 tsp. water
   ½ tsp. lemon extract

Measure out oil phase into medium-size enamel pot and melt together slowly over boiling water. Then take off source of heat, and allow to cool to *warm*. The mixture must remain completely fluid, but needn't be any hotter than that.

Meanwhile measure out the water phase, and mix thoroughly. *Do not heat.*

Add the water phase to the oil phase *slowly,* stirring *by hand* enough to make sure that the oil phase accepts the water phase completely. The best way is to add a bit of the water phase, stir it in, then add another bit, and so on. After the water phase is completely stirred into the oil phase, whip the entire mixture with your electric beater on *high* for about a minute. Spoon into jars. Makes a bit less than a cup of rich, pale-gold, lemony cream.

LEMON CREAM is a natural pH cosmetic; that is, it's slightly acid (due to the presence of lemon juice), and thus helps the skin maintain its normal pH, which is slightly acid, about 5.5. It's elegant as a rich night cream,

as a dry area cream, or for use anywhere that your skin
needs some special conditioning and t.l.c. It's beautifully
moisturizing, due to the whopping amount of lanolin;
emollient, thanks to mineral oil and petrolatum; and it
smells *absolutely marvellous* (especially if the lemon juice
is fresh!)

If you're adventuresome, try substituting other fruit
juices for the lemon juice—especially citrus. Or try various
vegetable juices, alone or with lemon juice, perhaps carrot
or cucumber, and take advantage of their vitamin content
as well as their natural acidity.

But just plain LEMON CREAM is such a golden beauty
that you'd better memorize the recipe. You'll find yourself
making it again and again. I must confess (though perhaps I shouldn't play favorites) that of all Dr. T.'s master-
creams, *I* like this one best!

A word of caution, though: *all* acid pH creams and
lotions are *heaven* for molds and microbes. So be sure to:

Label: Keep Refrigerated!

CHERRY HAND LOTION

Oil phase:
   3 tbsp. lanolin
   1 tbsp. petrolatum (petroleum jelly)
   1 tbsp. mineral oil
   1 tbsp. solid vegetable shortening
              or
   ¼ cup plus 2 tbsp. MOTHER BASE #4
      (*see* Mother Bases)

  and

Water phase:
   2 tbsp. glycerine
   ¼ cup plus 2 tbsp. 10% SOAP STOCK
      (*see* Base Stocks)
   1 cup water

2 tbsp. SUSPENSION JELLY (*see* Base Stocks)
6 drops red food color
1 tsp. cherry flavoring or cherry extract

Measure oil phase into medium size enamel pot and heat over boiling water until quite hot—*not* boiling.

Meanwhile, heat the water phase separately until everything is dissolved together, and it, too, is quite hot.

Do not beat either phase. *Hand stir only.*

Add the water phase to the oil phase, with *hand stirring.* Then pour (through funnel) into a pretty bottle. Since this makes about two cups (sixteen ounces), the bottle will have to be fairly large. (If you're planning to use several small bottles, pour the mixture *at this point* into a large jar, continue cooling and mixing, and when it's finished, *shake it thoroughly,* then decant into smaller bottles.)

Now add the food color and cherry flavor, and, *holding the bottle under cold running water,* swirl and shake gently to thoroughly mix the contents. If you see foam developing on top, carefully skim or pour it off. Continue to swirl and bathe in cool water until lotion is room temperature.

This makes a mild, rich hand lotion with a lovely fragrance. (You can use other flavorings, and change the name to fit. Apricot is one of our favorites; also almond extract or rose soluble perfume oil. Be daring!)

If you haven't made up SUSPENSION JELLY, you *can* leave it out, but the product will tend to feel a bit thin, and require shaking up before each use. Its soothing, smoothing qualities, though, will be unimpaired. Keep a bottle by your kitchen sink for after-dishes hand-pampering; in fact, why not give it a *color and fragrance* to go with your kitchen decor? (In fact, why not keep a bottle by your *bathroom* sink, and give it a color and fragrance to match your *bathroom* decor? And if you have *two* bathrooms . . . !)

YUM-YUM APRICOT pH LOTION

1 tsp. pectin (dry powder)
2 tsp. glycerine
1 tsp. solid vegetable shortening
¼ cup fresh lemon juice (strained) or
   reconstituted
¼ cup plus 2 tbsp. water
1 drop red food coloring
¼ tsp. apricot flavoring

Measure the shortening and glycerine into a medium-size enamel pot and melt them together over hot water. Then work in the powdered pectin, using your electric mixer on *low*.

Meanwhile heat the water and lemon juice the same way, and when they reach a simmer, slowly add them, a little at a time, to the oil phase, beating constantly.

Remove from heat, and let cool. Stir your mixture by hand every now and then just to make sure it doesn't separate.

When it's cool, put it into a pretty bottle, and add the food coloring and apricot flavoring. Shake well. Makes about three-fourths cup of the most elegant, silken, yummy-smelling lotion imaginable—one of Dr. T.'s special triumphs! (The scientist in Dr. T. frowns unhappily at our frivolous title for what *he* imaginatively calls "Acid pH Hand-Body Lotion." But we couldn't help it! One sniff of this scrumptious liquid and we went utterly ape! And where did the idea for the apricot fragrance come from? Dr. T., on the prowl for new cosmeticook ideas, caught a whiff of the marvellous stuff his wife—a Viennese lady—keeps around for making those heavenly chocolate cakes. And was inspired!)

YUM-YUM APRICOT pH LOTION (a wince from Dr. T.) *is* yum-yum—but it has a more serious and useful purpose. As we all know, when our skin gets older it loses its ability to *do* certain things, like bending supple-y without wrinkling, or producing oil to lubricate itself. It also loses its knack of returning to its normal pH level. And about now is the time to explain what, in fact, pH *is*.

In laymen's (*our*) terms pH is the degree of acidity or alkalinity measurable in anything. For example, pH 7.0 is absolutely neutral. Any pH below 7.0 is acid; any pH above it is alkaline. The normal pH level of our skin is about 5.5, that is, slightly acid. A strong acid, like sulfuric acid, which will actually *char* the skin, has a pH of 1 to 2. At the other end of the scale, a strong alkali (another word for this is "caustic") like lye, with a pH of 12 or more, will burn, too. Since alkalis and acids are opposites, one will neutralize the other (which is why, for example, you might take a bit of baking soda—alkaline—in water to help an "acid stomach" kind of indigestion, or you might rinse off a strong caustic cleaning agent, like ammonia, with vinegar, an acid).

Most soaps and cosmetic creams are alkaline. *Young* skin has the ability to readjust its pH to normal acidity, but older skin often suffers skin fatigue; it just can't make it back home again, and gets dry, tired, and old looking. Hence the need, nay yearning, for a pH lotion that's slightly acid and nourishing and nondrying, to help the skin do its job of maintaining its pH level at 5.5. It's the lemon juice in this one that does the pH job; you should by now know the functions of the other ingredients by heart!

Incidentally, our cosmetic chemist furnishes some interesting side information: following the pH story down, since hair and skin are quite similar in composition (both are forms of the protein known as *keratin;* hair—and nails —are hard keratin, while skin is a softer version), they're also similar in the way they react to chemicals. So permanent waves are actually strongly alkaline hair *softeners* (around pH 9.5), which are carefully formulated to act on the hair so it can be reshaped into a curl, then neutralized and set into its new shape. If you go a little higher in pH, to about 11.5, the hair simply dissolves completely—and— presto!—you have a depilatory. And all with the same chemicals!

Note, though: all acid pH formulas are quick to grow mold, so be sure to:

Label: Keep Refrigerated.

CHAPTER THIRTEEN

SPECIALTIES OF THE HOUSE

ANTIPERSPIRANT CREAM

Oil phase:
    3 tbsp. lanolin
    1 tbsp. petrolatum (petroleum jelly)
    2 tbsp. solid vegetable shortening
                    or
    ¼ cup plus 1 tbsp. MOTHER BASE #3
        (*see* Mother Bases)

and

    2 tbsp. cocoa butter

and

Water phase:
    1 tbsp. glycerine
    1 tbsp. 10% SOAP STOCK (*see* Base Stocks)
    3 tbsp. water
    3 drops green food color
and

Antiperspirant solution:
    ¼ cup plus 1 tbsp. of 25% aluminum chloride
        solution (sold in most major drugstores,
        sometimes as "deodorant solution")

Measure oil phase together into a medium-size enamel
pot and heat over boiling water until *very hot*.

Meanwhile, measure water phase ingredients into a small enamel pot and heat until simmering. *Do not boil,* as it will foam over and make an awful mess.

Carefully add water phase to oil phase, stirring constantly with electric beater on *high.* Continue to whip away for about twenty seconds, then stop and let the foam come to the top of the mixture, skim it off, and remove mixture from heat.

Now let the mixture cool, hand stirring from time to time. To speed this process you can put the whole mixture, pot and all, into a large pan of *cold* water, but if you do, keep stirring and scraping down sides of pan so it won't cool with gunky lumps. Your object now is to stir it and cool it into a uniform light green water/oil *lotion.*

When the lotion is thoroughly cool, start adding the antiperspirant solution, *one-half teaspoon at a time,* beating constantly with your electric beater on *high.* This will take plenty of patience and time. *Don't rush it,* or the whole batch can invert (curdle) and an awful mess it is! The lotion now thickens dramatically as you add the antiperspirant solution, and forms a soft cream as you stir.

When all the antisperspirant solution is accepted by your cream, whip the whole batch for about two minutes with your electric mixer on *high.*

When you're finished, you'll have a lovely, non-tacky cream which is *very* effective. It has a somewhat sweet cocoa-butter fragrance, but can be perfumed, if you like. If you *do* like, try one-half teaspoon rose soluble perfume oil, or any perfume of your choice. Makes about one and one-half cups.

Any antiperspirant, including this one, can be rough on sensitive skin. So if you *are* sensitive, or show any signs of irritation at all—discomfort, slight redness or rash—discontinue use. Some people are very sensitive to these products, others not at all. This particular recipe, though effective, is relatively mild, with many soothing oils in the base, and shouldn't give trouble to anyone who doesn't normally react to other antiperspirants.

SOFT-SKIN ROLLING LOTION

Oil phase:
  2 tsp. lanolin
  1 tsp. solid vegetable shortening
  4 tsp. paraffin wax

Water phase:
  2 tbsp. 10% SOAP STOCK (*see* Base Stocks)
  ¼ cup water
  1 tbsp. SUSPENSION JELLY (*see* Base Stocks)

Measure out ingredients of oil phase into a small enamel pan and heat until *very hot* over boiling water. Remove from heat.

Meanwhile, heat the water phase as well, being careful *not* to boil, as SOAP STOCK will foam over.

Now add the water phase to the molten wax and oils and *hand stir.* As the mixture begins to cool, it will begin to thicken a bit. At first it will want to separate the minute you stop stirring, but after awhile it will begin to hold together. Now get out the electric beater, and beat at *medium* speed for one minute only. Then spoon off the foam that forms on top, and continue to stir *by hand* until the mixture cools to hand warm.

At this point, bottle your mixture. You'll have a bit over a half cup. Cap the bottle, and shake the still-warm lotion from time to time, letting it cool slowly the rest of the way.

You'll have a rich, creamy white lotion when thoroughly cooled. Now for the ultimate test! Unscrew the cap and try a bit on the back of your hand. Rub . . . rub . . . rub . . . and presto! The emulsion breaks as the water evaporates, and out pops the wax. A bit more rubbing makes little *balls* of it, little balls that *roll around* and pick up anything loose that they encounter—dead skin, soil, scales, whatever. Then just brush or rinse off the *rolling* balls of wax, and your skin is clean, de-scaled, and baby-soft.

The trick in making a ROLLING LOTION is to use waxes rather than oils, and to make an emulsion that's stable enough to look pretty (and stay together) in the bottle, yet not *too* stable, so it will fall apart readily as you rub it on. Our cosmetic chemist did this one with a special niceness. He used—with his own brand of humor—lanolin, an *animal* product (sometimes known as "wool wax" in the trade), solid shortening, a *vegetable* product, and paraffin, a *mineral* wax: animal, vegetable, and mineral— and no oils at all, since they would soften and dilute the waxy materials so that the lotion wouldn't roll up properly. For an emulsifier, Dr. T. chose good old SOAP STOCK —just enough to keep the emulsion together—plus a bit of SUSPENSION JELLY just to hold things together. A masterful formula, and one that Dr. T. preens himself over unbearably (but with justice).

Try SOFT-SKIN ROLLING LOTION on callused feet, grey, tough-skinned elbows, scaly backs of hands—anywhere that dead or callused skin uglifies you. And miracle of miracles, it vacuums up that dead dry stuff like your mama's old upright. Dr. T., we salute you!

WATERLESS HAND CLEANER

    1 tbsp. paraffin wax
    1 tbsp. solid vegetable shortening
    ¼ cup light mineral oil
    2 tbsp. 10% SOAP STOCK (*see* Basic Stocks)

Measure wax, shortening and mineral oil into a small enamel pan and heat over boiling water until quite hot. Remove from heat when completely melted.

Then add the (cool) SOAP STOCK in a steady stream to the oil mixture, beating constantly with your electric mixer on *medium*.

The mixture will whiten and thicken (you know what an emulsion looks like by now). Scoop up into a jar, and set aside to cool. Makes about one-half cup of firm white cream.

This isn't exactly a cosmetic, but it's fun to make and have around for hubby when he operates on the car engine or gets creative down in the shop. And it works as well— and smells a whole lot better!—than those solvent-y ones you buy and then worry about Junior getting into.

The term "waterless cleanser" is a misnomer; *all* of these products have water *in* them, which is why they can live up to their claim of not needing water to help them do their work. All you do is work WATERLESS into greasy hands, wait a minute or two, then wipe it off. The mineral oil is the ingredient that does most of the work in loosening grime, grease, paint. WATERLESS liquefies the minute you rub it on, and turns from a cream to a thin, guck-removing film which can be wiped off with nothing rougher than a paper tissue when its job is done. It hates and repels water, but even the soapiest water won't work on grease the way *this* does. And if your hands—and your husband's—just don't get grimy, try WATERLESS as a lubricant for moving metal parts, or a grease cleanser in the kitchen or the garage. You'll be surprised and delighted!

FOUNDATION BASE

2 tbsp. BEESWAX BASE (*see* Base Stocks)

or

    1 tbsp. beeswax
    1 tbsp. safflower oil

and

3 tbsp. SUSPENSION JELLY (*see* Base Stocks)

and

    ¼ cup glycerine
    ½ cup 10% SOAP STOCK (*see* Base Stocks)
    4 tsp. 70% *ethanol* rubbing alcohol

Measure out beeswax and safflower oil (or BEESWAX

BASE) plus glycerine into medium size enamel pot and melt together over boiling water. Stir by hand until the mixture is perfectly smooth, and wax is completely dissolved.

Meanwhile heat (direct heat is all right here) SOAP STOCK to very hot, well above a simmer. *Don't boil,* or it will foam over and make a horrible mess. Watch it carefully, and heat until it thins out and *wants* to foam.

Remove the first mixture from the heat carefully.

Now *slowly,* stirring by hand only enough to avoid foam, add the SOAP STOCK to the mixture of wax and oils. After you mix the two, add the SUSPENSION JELLY and, as you keep stirring and cooling, the batch will whiten and thicken somewhat.

Set the batch aside and allow to cool, stirring occasionally, until hand warm. Then add the rubbing alcohol and stir in thoroughly. Bottle. Makes about a cup and a quarter.

If the FOUNDATION BASE becomes uncomfortably gelled after a few days, one or two teaspoons more of alcohol can be worked in to thin it to the consistency you like best. But don't let it get too thin, or it won't hold your powder in suspension when you make LIQUID MAKEUP.

FOUNDATION BASE *can* be used as is, with loose powder applied over it. But by far the favorite use for such a base is *with* the powder worked in, as in LIQUID MAKEUP.

LIQUID MAKEUP

¼ cup FOUNDATION BASE
4 tsp. face powder

Choose a face powder that's fine in texture and is the world's best color for you, as it will act as the coloring agent for this makeup.

Work the powder into the FOUNDATION BASE by hand, using a spoon or spatula. The color of the powder may darken or "develop" when it hits the base, but you'll find that it will come back to more or less its original color when the MAKEUP you're compounding dries on your skin.

When the powder is all wetted out into the base, scoop the mixture up onto the flat part of a china plate and grind with the back of the spoon or the spatula blade. Add a few drops of alcohol (or vodka) if it's too thick.

After it's all uniformly ground and lovely, take an old, clean nylon stocking and carefully force your MAKEUP through the toe. It will emerge beautifully refined and filtered and ready-to-wear.

LIQUID MAKEUP—TEEN-AGE STYLE

¼ cup LIQUID MAKEUP
1 to 2 tsp. calamine lotion

Simply add one to two teaspoons of the calamine lotion (your druggist will supply it for pennies if you don't have some around the house already) to the LIQUID MAKEUP, and mix thoroughly.

The calamine lotion is *very* kind to teen-age oily skin bumps, and the zinc oxide and bentonite (white clay) suspended therein help give the makeup extra covering power, to hide those nasty reds. The color of the calamine *may* change the MAKEUP color a bit, so if you *know* you're going to be compounding the teen-age variety, you can make allowances from the beginning, and test out your powder *plus* calamine for color, before you go the whole way with the FOUNDATION BASE formula. No reason you couldn't also (provided you know when you start cooking up FOUNDATION BASE, that the batch will be for teen-age use) add a bit (one-fourth cake) of USP camphor, crumbled, to the alcohol in the FOUNDATION BASE recipe. This will give a nice bit of extra zing and pimple power to the final product.

VELVET PAWS FOOT POWDER

2 tbsp. boric acid (get the finely powdered grade)
½ cup talc
½ cup corn starch
½ tsp. peppermint extract
1 tsp. rubbing alcohol (either kind okay here)

First dry-blend the three powders by putting them in your blender, and giving them a thorough going-over on *high;* or put them in a large, clean, dry, *closeable* jar and shake them up together.

Then, separately, mix the peppermint extract (for its cooling menthol content) and the alcohol and, using an empty window cleaner spray bottle or atomizer, *spray* them into the powder mixture, either while the blender is going, or—if you used the jar method—a tiny bit at a time, shaking well after each spray. If you have *no* spray bottle or atomizer available, use an eyedropper, but shake or blend very thoroughly, so that the liquid is completely mixed into the powder combination.

This is a lovely, aromatic, absorbent foot powder, delicious to apply after baths. It's soothing, cooling, and mildly antiseptic.

CHAPTER FOURTEEN

WHAT IS A SUNTAN LOTION?

Ideally, a suntan lotion is one that screens out nearly all of the burning rays of the sun, and lets the tanning ones through. The problem is in proportions. If the objective is a beautiful, lasting tan, *all* the tanning rays possible should be allowed to reach the skin, plus *some* burning rays, because without that little "kicker" of burning rays, the tan that develops will be a transient one that develops about twelve hours after exposure and is already beginning to fade after four or five days. The true, lasting tan takes several days to develop fully, and then *stays around* for four or five *months* before it fades completely. But if *too* many burning rays hit the skin, it may blister and peel, thereby messing up whatever tan you've patiently acquired. So the cosmetic chemist's job is to *balance* the burning and tanning rays and come up with a product that gives the most true tan and the least burn possible.

Actually sunscreens are a relatively new invention. The first ones were introduced in the 'twenties, and in World War II, the Navy enthusiastically adopted the idea and equipped all its lifeboats with "Red Vet Pet" (red veterinary petrolatum), a water-repellent, greasy, awful stuff which saved many a sailor from a bad sunburn, but actually screens less efficiently than an elegant modern cosmetic like WHIPPED SUNTAN.

The term "sun*tan* lotion" is actually a misnomer. Nothing except the sun will make you tan. There *are* stainers on the market which actually color the skin. These have had a vogue lately as "after shave bronzers" (the man of the house likes to look virilely tan, too) but they're basically the same as the leg tans you used to cover your early-summer whiteness a few years back, and they're first cousins to the leg makeup now coming back into style. Most of these stainers have the unpleasant habit of rubbing off on chairs and skirts when they get wet—no substitute for a true, on-you suntan. You may have also run into the indoor-outdoor suntan product, which contains both DHA (a chemical which turns brownish after about four or five hours' contact with the amino acids of the skin) and a good sunscreen which allows you to expose yourself to the sun and develop a real tan while sporting an ersatz DHA one.

WHIPPED SUNTAN

Oil phase:
   ¼ cup lanolin
   ¼ cup sesame oil

Water phase:
   ¾ cup water
   3 tea bags

Heat the water to boiling and soak the three tea bags in it, squeezing occasionally, for twenty minutes. Remove the tea bags. What's left is about one-half cup of quadruple strength tea.

In another medium-size enamel pot, measure out the lanolin and sesame oil, and heat them gently over boiling water.

As soon as the oil phase is melted together, take it out of the hot water and *slowly* add the one-half cup strong tea, beating constantly with your electric mixer on *medium*. Pour the tea slowly, in a thin stream, and watch carefully, making sure that the emulsion accepts the tea. If it doesn't, and some tea appears to be floating on top of the lotion which is forming, *stop adding tea* for a bit and keep beating until all the tea is absorbed. Then begin *slowly* to pour again. Continue this process until all the tea is used.

Finally, when all the tea has been accepted into the lotion, increase your beater speed to *high* and fluff the cream by actually whipping it for three to four minutes. During this final whip, you can perfume if you like by adding about one-half teaspoon of a fragrance you like.

You've now made about one cup of a lovely, soft tan (cafe au lait) colored cream which spreads beautifully on the skin, gives a superb moist sensation as it rubs in, and then dries without a sign of tackiness. It is a true absorption base—a water/oil cream which is actually water *repellent* (spread a bit on a clean spatula, add a drop or two of water, and try to mix them; you can't). What a lovely quality for beach or sunbathing; the water repellency makes SUNTAN *stay on* through sweating and swimming—or at least a reasonable amount of same.

As for its sun-taming ability, SUNTAN will screen out about half of the erythemal rays of the sun (meaning rays which turn the skin red, ergo "burning") but will allow almost 90 percent of the *tanning* rays to get through. It's *not* a total sunscreen, and not intended for those super-fair blondes who get burned after five minutes of beach exposure; if you're one, you'll want to protect your skin with one of the highly efficient sun-blocking products which are on the market commercially. However SUNTAN is a lovely cream for hardier skins, and can even be made more efficient (and darker-looking) by increasing the number of tea bags in the original strong tea solution. So throw away that baby oil, toss out that old 'thirties home-mixed remedy, iodine and baby oil, and whip up some SUNTAN.

Why is what's in it in it? Dr. T. elucidates: Tea is a rich source of tannins and tannic acid (the dark coloring matter in tea as well as in various barks and roots). And tannic acid, you may remember, is an excellent burn remedy, as well as a mild sunscreen. Didn't your mama keep a tube of tannic acid jelly on the shelf above her stove for soothing burns and scalds? Mine did! She claimed—and Dr. T. confirms—that if it's used fast enough, it may even keep burn scars from developing. Sesame oil has the highest ultraviolet absorbance of all the natural oils, due to its high polyunsaturate content. And our old and good friend lanolin is, as you surely know by now, a rich, emollient absorption base (water loving, therefore holds moisture to the skin) emulsifier. So . . . !

In case you're wondering about shortcuts, Dr. T. makes a note on SUNTAN that should interest you; he tried *instant tea* in one variation of the SUNTAN formula and found it wasn't nearly as good—probably because the (bitter tasting) tannins are largely removed in the "instant-izing"; what's left gives *only half the sun-screening power*.

CHAPTER FIFTEEN

BASE STOCKS AND MOTHER BASES

Certain combinations of ingredients in cosmeticookery (like certain combinations in culinary cookery) are used together so often that they're like Heavenly Twins—if you see one, you're pretty sure the other isn't far behind. It behooves you, then, if you're really going to practice cosmeticookery as an art, to find ways of precombining some of these elements (and sometimes they come in threes and fours as well) to save time in the preparation of your beauty jams and jellies, and also because sometimes (as with the waxes and oils) they're easier to handle in combination than they are apart.

These Base Stocks, then, are *examples* of ways in which you can put together, for future use, elements that appear together often in your cosmetic recipes. The BEESWAX and PARAFFIN WAX BASES are *much* easier to measure out and melt than either beeswax or paraffin wax alone. So in *any* recipe that calls for one of these waxes *plus* an oil (*any* oil) you can merely measure out *double* that amount of base (subtracting the extra from the *oil* called for) and proceed, secure in the knowledge that you've gotten everything called for into the recipe, and saved yourself a bit of trouble in the bargain. (See NOURISHING CREAM recipe for an example of how this is done.)

But don't stick to the examples we've given. *Every* housewife has probably mixed up a shaker jar of cinnamon and sugar in her day, or maybe one of salt, pepper, garlic powder, MSG, and paprika, as a barbeque salt.

Same principle. You might find you especially like to use rose soluble perfume oil with red food color; mix up a batch. Or do the same with peppermint extract and green, or green-blue. The principle works best with long-life ingredients, but if you get in the habit of thinking in terms of bases, you'll be surprised at the many *variations* that present themselves to you. And it may encourage you to experiment with more abandon, not only on what you put *into* the bases, but on what you put *around* them.

Mother bases are a special breed of pussycat because they embody the active *heart* of a recipe. Everything else in a recipe is more or less window dressing; the Mother is the thing that carries the freight.

If you understand that principle, and study the Mother bases given here, you should be able to come up with almost infinite varieties of creams and lotions—substituting as *you* like for the other ingredients, varying texture, color, fragrance, emolliency, moisturizing ability, skin-feel, vitamin content, whatever—as *you* choose. And that's one of the major purposes of this book: to help you to be *creative* in your cosmeticookery, and make custom products, *to your taste,* that you couldn't possibly find among the welter of mass-produced goodies for sale.

10% SOAP STOCK
(Fondly known as "Soap Soup")

1 oz. avoirdupois *pure* soap flakes

for each

1 cup water

Heat water to a simmer *(don't boil!)* and add soap flakes. Stir till clear. Bottle and keep. SOAP STOCK may go cloudy, gelatinous, or even curdly when cool. That's all right. Just shake it up and rewarm it till clear before you use it. "Soap soup" will keep for many months, and need not be refrigerated.

Notice, please, that the above directions, *contrary to any others in this book,* call for a *weight* ounce, not a *fluid* ounce of soap flakes. If you don't have a reliable kitchen scale, buy the smallest possible box of soap flakes, read the net contents (in avoir ounces), dump the whole box in a large pot and add one cup of water for each ounce. You'll have lots of soap soup—but there are lots of ways you can use it.

Notice, also, please, that soap flakes come in a variety of forms, highly fluffed, mixed with detergents, all detergent, with added softeners or enzymes or bluing or borax, etc. *Don't use any such!* Find one which clearly states *pure soap flakes,* like the one you know and we know and our mamas knew, and *all* of us used for baby things. That's the one we used in all the formulas in this book.

BEESWAX BASE

¼ cup beeswax
¼ cup safflower oil

Measure safflower oil into one- or two-cup Pyrex measuring cup. Chip pieces of beeswax into the oil until the level reaches one-half cup; you've now chipped in one-fourth cup beeswax. (*That's* a technique the housewife taught the cosmetic chemist!)

Now set the measuring cup into boiling water and stir carefully until the oil and the wax melt together and dissolve into one liquid.

Pour into a jar and let cool. You now have a soft paste which is *much* easier to measure and melt than the beeswax alone. Just remember, this is not a substitute for beeswax; it's a substitute for beeswax *plus* an equal amount of oil. Study the recipe for NOURISHING CREAM, for instance, and you'll see what we mean.

PARAFFIN WAX BASE

¼ cup paraffin wax ("household" wax,
  used for sealing jams and preserves)
¼ cup light mineral oil

Measure the mineral oil into a one or two-cup Pyrex measuring cup and chip the wax into the oil until the level reaches one-half cup (as for BEESWAX BASE).

Now place the Pyrex cup over boiling water and heat until wax and oil melt and dissolve together. Then jar the mixture and let cool. As with BEESWAX BASE, you now have a mixture that's much easier to measure and melt than paraffin alone.

SUSPENSION JELLY

2 tsp. dry cornstarch
1 tbsp. water
¼ cup glycerine

Stir all ingredients together without heating. Then place in a small enamel pot and heat (direct heat is all right here) until the mixture suddenly thickens to a pudding-like consistency (just before it reaches the boiling point). Remove from heat, jar while still hot, and seal.

The purpose for SUSPENSION JELLY is threefold: it helps hold emulsions together; it improves and thickens texture, and it keeps color pigments suspended in emulsions (as in makeups and foundation bases). The cosmetic industry has a gaggle of intricate emulsifiers and gums available to do these things, but the home cosmeticook has to use what she can get, be ingenious with what drug and art and grocery stores have to offer her. SUSPENSION JELLY *is* ingenious, and, what's more, is an admirable substitute for the more complex substances used in the trade to do the same jobs. (This will keep at room temperature and need not be refrigerated.)

MOTHER BASE #1,

or

LECITHIN BASE

1 egg yolk
1 tbsp. glycerine
1 tbsp. castor oil

Simply beat the ingredients together, without heat, until smooth. Bottle. Shake before using.

A tiny bit of this base, used in a recipe with witch hazel or alcohol, tends to make the effect of the alcohol less drying. Since it's such a superb *ingredient* in rich creams and lotions, why not dab it, *straight,* on problem skin areas? It's a gorgeous emollient, full of vitamins, and has a beautiful feel on the skin.

Because this is a base and not a finished cosmetic, it may tend to separate a bit on standing. Just shake, shake before using.

MOTHER BASE #2,

or

LANOLIN-COCOA BUTTER BASE

1 tbsp. lanolin
1 tbsp. cocoa butter
¼ cup plus 2 tbsp. sesame oil

Measure ingredients into small enamel pot and melt together over boiling water. Make sure all fats are clearly dissolved. Stir. Jar. Set aside to cool. Makes one-half cup.

This base may cloud somewhat on cooling, but won't separate, and is just as good cloudy as clear, so long as the fats were thoroughly mixed to begin with. It's an ingredient in other products, but also a luscious *cleansing oil* all by itself. Try it for removing dirt or grease from *you,* or from furniture, leather, or metal. It works!

Now try a little experiment, to increase your cosmeti-cookability:

First, put a drop or two of plain sesame oil on the back of your hand and try to rub it in. It doesn't go, really. There's always a faintly greasy feeling. But don't take our word for it, please. Do it yourself, and get the feel.

Now try the same with MOTHER BASE #2. Feel the difference! The lanolin and cocoa butter have completely changed the feel of the sesame oil, and MOTHER BASE #2 leaves a protective layer on the skin that's much drier, not greasy at all. Perhaps "waxy" would be a good word for MOTHER BASE #2's personality; in any case, it's not hard to take at all.

Finally, let's go one step further, and make an *emulsion* of our beautiful MOTHER BASE. Put three tablespoons of it in a small bottle and add (cold; just plop it in) one tablespoon water. Then *shake hard.* An emulsion will form promptly; it's not a finished formulation, not stabilized, so it will fall apart in an hour or two, but *feel it.* It's the same oil, and the water will evaporate from your skin a few minutes after you rub it in, but *feel* the difference! It's now *rich* on the skin as you apply it, and distinctly less oily. Enrobing the oil droplets in water makes *all* the difference!

This little "feelie" experiment shows the dramatic difference between oils and emulsions—and the *value* of emulsions in cosmetic formulas. Thank you, Dr. Galen! (If this mystifies you, see CLEANSING CREAM FOR NORMAL SKIN.)

Incidentally, the emulsion you just formed can be used to good effect as an emollient for dry skin or dry hair.

MOTHER BASE #3

3 tbsp. lanolin
1 tbsp. petrolatum (petroleum jelly)
2 tbsp. solid vegetable shortening

Measure all ingredients into a small enamel pot, melt over boiling water until thoroughly dissolved together, stir, and jar.

This is the "Mother of Creams," along with its almost-identical twin, MOTHER BASE #4, below.

MOTHER BASE #4

3 tbsp. lanolin
1 tbsp. petrolatum (petroleum jelly)
1 tbsp. solid vegetable shortening
1 tbsp. mineral oil

Melt together, stir, and jar, as with MOTHER BASE #3.

MOTHER BASE #3 appears in our ANTIPERSPIRANT CREAM where it manages to hold things together in the presence of the very-difficult-to-emulsify deodorant solution, the antiperspirant active ingredient.

MOTHER BASE #4 is the heart of my favorite of favorites. It is used in LEMON CREAM, again a problem child in emulsion terms, due to the *lemon juice,* which can easily curdle all sorts of emulsions—as you well know from adding it to tea and milk! And if it will accept and emulsify pure lemon juice, you *know* it will take any other juice you can dream up. So have a ball!

Anyone for borscht?

APPENDIX

INGREDIENTS

ALBUMIN—egg white. More accurately, albumin is a film-forming protein found *in* egg white. The albumin is about one-seventh of the total; the other six-sevenths are mostly water, which evaporates when you spread egg white on your face and leaves a gradually *tightening* feeling. Ergo—its use in facial masks and various astringent preparations. Also, it happens to be an excellent emulsion stabilizer—holding them together when they want to separate because you have added some exotic (incompatible) ingredient. Also, it contains essential amino acids, as do all proteins—good for the skin.

ALCOHOL—*see* RUBBING ALCOHOLS

ALMOND EXTRACT—available at most food stores. A food flavoring, generally made from bitter almonds and often fortified with synthetic flavorings. Excellent as a *perfume* for cosmetics.

ALUMINUM CHLORIDE SOLUTION—available in some large chain drug stores as a *25 percent solution,* also usually labelled "deodorant solution." Ask your druggist to be sure. Do not merely ask for a deodorant or you will be handed any one of dozens of brand name products.

Aluminum Chloride was the first *antiperspirant* salt to be used for commercial products of this sort, and is still the strongest available—both in effectiveness and in acidity. It is also quite antiseptic, thus acting as a *deodorant* as well as an antiperspirant. Caution: can be irritating to sensitive skin. Discontinue use of *any* antiperspirants if signs of irritation develop.

ANISE—available at many food stores as anise extract, a food flavor which is quite interesting as a "masculine note" perfume ingredient for cosmetics.

ARABIC—*see* GUM ARABIC

AROMATIC BITTERS—available in food and liquor stores. *Aromatic* means that these bitters have a heady *aroma,* as well as the characteristic taste which is so prized for certain mixed drinks. Putting it more simply, aromatic bitters make an excellent addition to your home perfumery kit. A few shakes from the bottle will give your product a certain *heady warmth* to the fragrance.

BEESWAX—available from various sources: some drug stores, some arts and crafts hobby supply stores, from candle-makers and some plumbers' supply houses, and finally, of course, from those who raise bees for honey. One pound of beeswax is produced by bees (as the honeycomb) for each eight pounds of honey.

Beeswax (which is produced by *virgin* bees only) is specified as the only wax to be used in religious candles produced for the Catholic church. It is an *ester*-wax; chemically 80 percent of it is ceryl myristate, with a very high melting point. This feature, plus its ability to form an emulsifier when reacted with *borax,* makes it of greatest value in producing stiff, high sheen, very stable creams.

BENTONITE—available at arts and crafts stores, especially those with ceramic supplies.

A highly purified white clay (*montmorillonite,* found in the midwest U.S.A. and Canada) which is used in cosmetics to *thicken* lotions, to *suspend* makeup pigments, and in facial masks, to *absorb oil* on the face, thereby reducing shine, producing a matte finish. When mixed with about ten times its own weight of water, *swells* considerably.

BENZOIN—*see* TINCTURE OF BENZOIN

BORAX—available in all supermarkets (Soaps and Detergents section) as well as in many drug stores.

A mild (pH 9.5) alkali material, borax is found almost pure in huge natural deposits (alkali flats) in the Far West, notably in Death Valley, California. It is an excellent cleanser *per se* (reacting with fats and oils to form borate soaps) and—for the same reason—an excellent *emulsifier* for cosmetics. It is most often used to form *water in oil* (w/o) emulsions such as cold creams and rich night creams and treatment creams.

BORIC ACID, POWDERED—primarily available in drug stores, but also in some supermarkets in the drug section.

A mild antiseptic having both bactericidal and fungicidal properties, yet mild enough to be included in some eye wash lotions. Talcs and foot powders containing up to 10 percent powdered boric acid are considered safe, but the *pure* powder should not be used as a dusting powder, especially not for infants.

CAMPHOR, USP—available as ½ oz. cakes, individually wrapped in cellophane at most drug stores.

Originally, all camphor came from camphor trees in Java, China and Brazil. The trees had to be at least fifty years old before they produced this interesting material. Now, 75 percent of the world supply is made synthetically, in factories that are generally less than fifty years old! It is used in plastics, explosives and fireworks, and in the drug and cosmetic fields as a counterirritant and occasional skin anesthetic material. It contains significant quantities of *azulene,* an anti-inflammatory healing and soothing agent.

CAUTION! Do not use mothballs (paradichlorobenzene) where camphor is called for in cosmetic formulas. "Para" is *not* to be put on the skin and is *not* the same as camphor, even though camphor has also been used at times as a moth-preventative. Be sure to look for the *USP* label on camphor intended for skin application. This designation means suitable for use in U.S. pharmaceuticals.

CASTOR OIL—available at all drug stores.

This extremely valuable oil, expressed from the Castor bean, is also known as oil of *Palma Christi*—if that makes any of you feel better about using it.

Actually, its use internally as a purgative is one of the least important, from a commercial point of view. Huge quantities are used yearly in resins and fibers, in detergents, in polishes, in carbon paper and in cosmetics—where at least half the lipsticks sold in this country contain a substantial proportion of castor oil, as do many men's hair dressings.

Its value stems from the fact that it is a semi-*drying* oil, forming a tough, shiny film when exposed to the air. Also, it is polyunsaturated, an excellent solvent for lipstick "staining" dyes, and has excellent keeping qualities. Is is (curiously) somewhat alcohol soluble, but *not* soluble in mineral oil.

COCOA BUTTER—available in most drug stores.

Also known as "theobroma oil" from the fact that it (as well as cocoa itself) is obtained from roasted seeds of the *Theobroma cacao* plant. In an emergency, you *could* use "white chocolate" in your formulas in place of cocoa butter. Chocolate, after all, is primarily cocoa butter plus sugar; but use of chocolate leaves a "tacky" feel due to the sugar content—and also presents preservation problems.

Cocoa butter is a well-known lubricant for massage purposes, as well as a suppository base and is used in many soaps and creams as an emollient soft waxy base.

CORN OIL—available in all food stores.

Corn oil is one of the heaviest feeling of the common vegetable oils. It is also a semi-drying oil, thickening on exposure to air. It has a relatively high unsaturated fatty acid content, making it of interest for cosmetics as well as oleomargarines. (By the way—oleo is a w/o emulsion of water emulsified *into* corn oil or some other vegetable oil, using lecithin as a prime emulsifier, and having the peculiar property that a *measured amount of air* is emulsified into the mixture as well.)

CORNSTARCH—available at all food stores.

A polysaccharide. It serves as a *desiccant* (absorbing water) and as a *thickener* in cosmetics. Thus, it is often included in dusting powders and foot powders for the first property, and occasionally in makeup items to suspend the pigments, due to its thickening ability. Finally, starch acts as an "anti-pruritic" material—stopping simple itch from dry skin. It is therefore found in a number of dermatological products and bath preparations intended for this use.

Note: for several decades, *rice* starch was the basis of most face powders and the early pressed powders. It has now largely been replaced by other materials which are not subject to bacterial decomposition.

CUCUMBER JUICE—cucumbers may be growing in your back yard. If not, they are certainly available in your local food store. Always juice *fresh* cucumbers, *peel and all,* in your blender or juicer, to get the best yield of fragrance, color, and vitamins. Spoils quickly—keep the juice itself, and any cucumber cosmetics, in the refrigerator at all times. Feels cool and satiny; imparts a heavenly fragrance.

DEODORANT SOLUTION—*see* [25 PERCENT] ALUMINUM CHLORIDE

EGG—*see* LECITHIN (egg yolk), ALBUMIN (egg white). Note: one large egg = approximately one ounce (2 tbsp.).

ETHANOL—*see* RUBBING ALCOHOLS

EXTRACTS—*see* ALMOND, ANISE, LEMON, PEPPERMINT, RUM, TARRAGON, VANILLA

FOOD COLORS—available at many food stores as 1 to 2 percent solutions in dropper bottle sets of four or five basic colors. By all means, buy the set in such dropper bottles if at all possible; otherwise, get an eyedropper to use them. Most one-cup batches of cosmetics only require one or two *drops* of color to make them pleasing. Use color liberally—

except perhaps where you like the natural white or golden color of a cream. If you want to try *mixtures* of colors, better to premix and experiment in *water* first. It's also a good way to dilute your colors if necessary (how else can you measure out *half* a drop of color?).

(By the way, these food colors are certified—guaranteed by government test to be safe in any quantity used.)

GELATIN—*unflavored* gelatin is available at most food and drug stores. Flavored gelatins (for puddings and other desserts) generally contain large amounts of sugar, making them unsuitable for use in cosmetics.

Gelatin is obtained by boiling animal skin and bones (left over after dressing the meat for food purposes). It is the original gelling agent, a protein which is full of essential amino acids and which has been demonstrated to be substantive to hair—sticking to it (bodying it) even when applied *in a shampoo*. The obvious benefit: you can shampoo *out* the soil and shampoo *in* this superb conditioner and bodying agent. The result: a rash of protein-for-the-hair cosmetics have appeared in the past several years—most of them based on gelatin or its derivatives.

In other cosmetics, gelatin is used in peelable face masks (with glycerine) and as a fingernail strengthener.

GLYCERINE—available at all drug stores.

Glycerine is a very heavy, dense, sticky liquid, weighing 25 percent more than water for an equivalent volume, and having a sweet warm taste. It is about 60 percent as sweet as sugar. Its major use in cosmetics is as a *polyol humectant* —one of a group of substances which attract, absorb and *hold* moisture—thus keeping your cream soft even if the cap is left off accidentally, and keeping your skin moist when the cream is applied to it.

Glycerine is one of the most versatile of all chemical raw materials, finding use as a sweetener, as a solvent, as a humectant and skin emollient, in soaps, in antifreeze, in hydraulic jacks, as nitroglycerine in dynamite, in glues, and in 1574 other commercial uses quoted in a recent article!

And just to top the cake—it's a *natural* material, obtained as a by-product of soap manufacturing.

GUM ARABIC—available at some drug stores, hobby shops and botanical supply houses.

Gum Arabic, also known as *acacia gum,* is an exudate from several different acacia trees growing in the Sudan, Africa. Huge drops, called "tears," form on the branches and are picked off by workers at plantations set up for the purpose of harvesting this interesting material. It is insoluble in alcohol—as are most natural gums, but will dissolve in only twice its weight of water.

It is used to form various mucilages and jellies for pharmaceutical bases, and as the basis for certain types of candy. In cosmetics it serves as an emulsion stabilizer, to suspend pigments occasionally, and as a gelling agent. Painters occasionally use solutions of it as a fixative for pastels, and ceramists use it in their glazes to glue them to a piece prior to firing in kilns.

GUM KARAYA—available at botanical supply houses, some drug stores.

Also known as Indian tragacanth, it is the dried exudate from the *Sterculia urens* tree which grows in the central provinces of India. It is faintly acidic and much cheaper than tragacanth itself, hence its rather extensive use in textile printing pastes, in some foods, and in cosmetics.

It is unusual in swelling in 60 percent alcohol, in contrast to almost all other natural gums which (to the contrary) would be precipitated by such concentration. Thus, its prime cosmetic use is in finger wave lotions which dry quickly and are non-tacky.

GUM TRAGACANTH—availability: same as karaya and arabic gums.

Also a gummy exudate, this one from *Astragalus gummifer,* growing in Iran and Asia Minor. It is quite acidic, forming excellent gels which are used in pharmaceuticals, foods, candies, textiles and cosmetics. For best gel strength, do *not* heat, but let set in water for twenty-four hours. Tragacanth is one of the oldest drugs known to man.

IODINE—available as a *tincture* at all drug stores and many supermarkets.

Iodine tincture is perhaps the most familiar of all the common antiseptics used at home. Most of the commercial world supply comes from a Chilean nitrate-bearing earth called *caliche;* it is also purified from *seaweed.* Much of the common table salt consumed in this country is *iodized,* helping to prevent hyperthyroidism and goiter problems, just as *fluorinating* the water supply helps prevent tooth decay in growing children.

Iodine is a bactericide and fungicide (both) and one of the most potent antiseptics known to man. Pure, it is a bluish black metallic substance which has the peculiar property of *subliming,* that is, evaporating (as a corrosive, violet vapor) directly *from a solid to a gas.* Most materials are like water in this respect—they go from the *solid* (*ice* in the case of water) to the *liquid* stage when they melt, *and only from the liquid to the gas* (steam, in the case of water vapor).

Iodine is very reactive, chemically. It will react with all polyunsaturated fats and oils, being neutralized by them in the process of "iodinating" them. Therefore, don't expect to use it as a preservative where such oils are present. Also, it reacts with starch (gives a lovely blue color which you may have produced inadvertently on some child's starched clothing at times!).

ISOPROPANOL, ISOPROPYL ALCOHOL—*see* RUBBING ALCOHOLS

KARAYA—*see* GUM KARAYA

LANOLIN—available at all drug stores and in many supermarkets.

Lanolin (also known as wool fat or wool wax) is refined wool grease, the purified secretion product of the sebaceous glands of the sheep. We, too, have sebaceous glands and constantly exude a fatty material called *sebum,* chemically very similar to lanolin. Sebum causes oily skin and acne problems in puberty, but is generally extremely valuable to normal skin and hair health, acting as nature's own lubricant for them. A sebaceous gland is attached to the root of *each* hair on our bodies, for example, releasing just enough sebum (read, *lanolin*) to give it that lustrous healthy look as it grows out. Similarly, sebum (lanolin) makes the skin supple and coats any incipient scaliness to prevent that itchy sensation known as "dry skin."

Lanolin is obtained by simply *washing* raw wool, which has to be done before it can be spun into fibers anyhow. It is plentiful and cheap as a result. With all this going for it, no wonder it is used so universally in cosmetics!

The cholesterol derivatives in lanolin make it a marvellous *water-absorbing base* material, as well as an excellent natural emulsifier. This accounts for the *moisturizing* qualities of both our own sebum and the sheep's version, called lanolin. They absorb *and hold* water to the skin, giving it that dewy look.

LECITHIN—constitutes 8 to 9 percent of EGG YOLK.

Lecithin is a *phospholipid,* a natural emulsifier and spreading agent which is a cellular constituent of all life, both plant life and animals. For example, it is present in our brains as well as on our skin, in soy beans, in egg yolk. Because it complexes readily with proteins, it is a superb *emollient* material. It is soluble in alcohol and fats and oils. It is also a natural antioxidant for such fats, preventing their tendency to go rancid. It is occasionally used as a superfatting agent in soap bars, to make them less drying to the skin.

LEMON—the fresh fruit, juice and extract (flavor) are all generally available in food stores.

For cosmetic purposes, the so-called "reconstituted" grade of lemon juice is quite an adequate substitute for the fresh juice. If you use fresh, be sure to *strain* it carefully, to remove all pulp which would spoil the appearance of your cream or lotion.

Lemon juice contains 5 to 8 percent citric acid, a rather strong acid found in all citrus and many other fruits, which is used to adjust the pH of foods, in effervescent powders, to acidify soft drinks. It is *the* most commonly used acid in cosmetics—for cream rinses and hair color rinses, for astringents and some fresheners, for reducing the alkalinity of many products which would otherwise be irritating. It has been used as a home skin bleach (not too effective) as well.

Lemon extract, the perfume oil derived from the peel and then dissolved in alcohol, has been a favorite in cosmetics and home products for years.

MAGNESIUM CITRATE—available as a dilute solution at all drug stores.

This is the magnesium salt citric acid, sold (for internal use as a mild cathartic) in *solution* form in small soda pop bottles containing one dose. This solution forms rather stiff glossy films when left to dry. When diluted suitably, has been sold as a hair set or bodying agent.

MENTHOL—as part of PEPPERMINT EXTRACT, available at most food stores.

Everything is "mentholated" these days, containing traces of menthol for its pepperminty taste or cool feel or refreshing odor. It is a peculiar craze of Americans, one which permeates our whole civilization to the point where mentholated shaving creams have a lot of menthol and the "regular" types contain only a little bit. The reason? Quite simple, really. The stuff works. In this particular case, *razor burn* is a problem with many men, and a trace of menthol in his shaving cream tends to cure the problem magically, cooling his face.

Menthol, however, can be rather irritating if used in too large a quantity. When it does, it starts to *heat* the skin instead of cooling it. Also, a tiny bit of mentholated cosmetic in your eye will give curious alternate hot-cold flashes of sensation. So, our first advice is, *keep mentholated prod-*

ucts out of eyes. It is actually irritating, as well as just giving funny temperature flashes, thus finding use in body rub liniments which heat the skin due to such effects.

Menthol is sometimes known as "peppermint camphor" and (when not made synthetically) is obtained from natural peppermint perfume oil, constituting about 28 percent of this oil. Pure menthol crystals are quite beautiful—long white needles—but for home cosmeticookery we will content ourselves with using peppermint extract.

MERTHIOLATE—at most drug stores and supermarkets.

A common skin antiseptic which will tend to discolor creams and lotions to which it is added. Its drug name is *thimerosal;* it is a compound of mercury, reacted with a derivative of salicylic acid. Not stable in sunlight.

METHYL SALICYLATE—available only in drug stores.

Methyl "Sal" is perhaps more familiar to you as oil of wintergreen. It is also sometimes called sweet birch oil. A highly aromatic yellowish oily liquid, it is very slightly soluble in water, but readily miscible with alcohol.

It is used in perfumery and as a food flavor (especially for candies). Externally (at levels of 10 to 35 percent or more) it is used as a counterirritant, relieving pain in sore muscles because it can be absorbed through the skin.

CAUTION: Do not ingest. Keep away from children. Do not use otherwise than as directed.

MICROCRYSTALLINE WAX—*see* PARAFFIN

MILK—An emulsion of approximately 3.8 percent butterfat in water, stabilized by the additional presence of about 3 percent *casein* protein. Total solids are approximately 12 percent, a level typical of most hand lotions on the market in the U.S.A. The natural product is produced by many mammals native to this country, notably the *cow.* Synthetic duplications, available for special dietary purposes in most supermarkets, should preferably not be used in cosmetics calling for *milk.*

MINERAL OIL—available at most drug stores and super-markets. Buy the light or medium weights if faced with a choice, not the "heavy."

A mixture of liquid hydrocarbons derived from petro-leum. Known also as "white oil" due to its colorless ap-pearance. Should also be tasteless and odorless for cosmetic and pharmaceutic purposes. Mineral oil tends to stay *on top of* the skin when applied in a cosmetic base. It does not penetrate at all, therefore leaving a shiny surface film and a certain amount of "slip," both of which are desirable for many purposes, especially for hair products. It is one of the best makeup removers known, because it wets the pigments easily and floats them off the skin, and exactly because it does *not* penetrate. An emollient product should penetrate if possible; a cleansing product should not.

OILS—commonly used in cosmetics, some of which are discussed in this book are: avocado, castor, corn, cotton-seed, cod liver, mineral, peanut, safflower, sesame and soybean oils. Less frequently used have been exotic varieties such as peach kernel oil, shark oil and sweet almond.

PARAFFIN WAX—available in most supermarkets and hard-ware stores.

You may know it better as "household wax" or as jam-sealing wax or as home-canning wax. It is a *mineral* wax, being actually the portion of petroleum which causes it to be so thick and heavy. In refining crude oil to produce gasoline and ordinary grade lubricating oils, the paraffin is removed. It is quite useful in home cosmetics because it is easily melted over boiling water and is readily available. How-ever, it does not produce as hard a cream as will the so-called microcrystalline wax. Microcrystalline wax, also a mineral wax, is available at some art supply stores for carving. In the chemical trade it is known as *ozokerite*. Paraffin, being softer and *not* having a crystalline structure, produces creams without a firm structure. If you can buy some microcrystalline wax, by all means try it in some of the formulas calling for paraffin; you'll note a considerable improvement, but be sure you get the *white* wax.

PECTIN—available in many food stores, for making jellies.

Pectin has similar action to gelatin. It comes from various fruits, notably the apple peel (which is why you will get stiffer jellies by mixing apple in with other fruits). Chemically, it is not a protein, but rather, a mixture of *methoxylated polygalacturonic acids*. (Wow!) It is a very soothing compound, often used internally in pharmaceutical practice. Has been used in cosmetics for its gelling and thickening properties. Mildly acidic, like the skin.

PEANUT OIL—available at most food stores.

Peanut oil is usually a greenish-yellow oil with a very pleasant odor. Its composition and uses are similar to those of olive oil in foods, soaps, paints and cosmetics. It is fairly heavy and slippery, reasonably unsaturated; excellent in cosmetics for various night creams and treatment creams.

PEPPERMINT EXTRACT—*see* MENTHOL

PERFUMES—*see* special section on PERFUMING elsewhere.

Many *perfume oils* are available at either drug stores or food stores. Many drug stores will sell small quantities of perfume oils which they stock for their own use in compounding prescriptions, or, they are willing to *order* such from their distributor if requested. By this means you should be able to obtain such oils as rose soluble, sometimes better known as rosewater perfume, or rose geranium and others suggested in this book. Lavender and lilac are occasionally available at drug stores too.

Many food *flavor extracts* make excellent perfumes, such as vanilla, rum, almond, anise, etc. which are mentioned in our recipe section.

Finally, the most fun and creative thing is to extract your own perfume oils—from herbs such as tarragon (which gives a chypre type of fragrance) or from odd things such as tobacco and spices. See the Perfuming section for details of procedure.

PETROLATUM—(PETROLEUM JELLY) available at drug
stores and supermarkets.

By all means buy the best (whitest) grade you can find.
The yellowish or reddish varieties have a rather awful penetrating odor which will permeate your products and cannot
be covered by addition of perfume later.

Petroleum jelly is generally obtained from Pennsylvania
crude oils, as part of the refining process. It is a marvelous
lubricant and, when properly purified, quite bland tasting,
making its use in lipsticks possible (to give them shine). It
is also useful to prevent tackiness in some cosmetics by
adding a bit of "slip" to the cream.

ROSEWATER—see PERFUMES

RUBBING ALCOHOLS—available at all drug stores and
supermarkets.

Most often, if you simply ask for "rubbing alcohol" without specifying which type, you will be handed the 70 percent ISOPROPYL ALCOHOL type. It is the most common,
and indeed, many stores will not carry any other. However, certain chain drug stores do carry the 70 percent
ETHANOL (or it may be called 70 percent ETHYL
ALCOHOL) type. There is a huge difference between them.
Each has uses in cosmetics.

ISOPROPYL ALCOHOL (sometimes called ISOPRO-
PANOL) is the better solvent of the two, dissolving various
oils easily. Also it is distinctly more irritating, thus really
stimulating the skin when rubbed on. Finally, it has a very
distinct odor which makes it absolutely unsuitable for use
in products which are to have a delicate fragrance—such as
astringents, skin fresheners, colognes and perfumes. Exception: when the desired stimulation is more important
than the fragrance.

ETHANOL is the alcohol meant when cosmetic formulas
call for alcohol without specifying which. It was used for
all of the perfume and flavor extracts which you have ever
smelled in your life. It is the drinking alcohol found in all
whiskies and liqueurs. (Although the ethanol sold in drug
stores for rubbing purposes has had a bitter material added,

to make it undrinkable; otherwise you would have to pay approximately $1.60 tax for each pint of rubbing alcohol!)

If you cannot find a source of ethanol rubbing alcohol, you can substitute *vodka* for it in these formulas. Vodka is only about 45 to 50 percent ethanol (90 to 100 proof), compared to the 70 percent (140 proof) strength of the rubbing alcohol. This will make a difference in your products, giving them less zing when applied to the skin, and also you may have trouble dissolving perfume oils in such weak alcohol. Most perfumes require *at least* 70 percent alcohol; some commercial products are as high as 85 percent (170 proof!) alcohol.

NOTE: by U.S. law, vodka contains *no* added flavor. Just alcohol and water.

SAFFLOWER OIL—available at most food and health stores.

Note the label on most bottles of safflower oil: "Rich in polyunsaturates" appears in one way or another, with various statements or implications of how such oil is healthful and necessary for life. This is so. Of all the common edible oils, safflower is the richest in *linoleates,* the chemical name for one of several essential fatty unsaturates.

The presence of these unsaturates makes safflower oil difficult to preserve (it tends to become rancid when kept too long, especially if it was not properly capped). This rancidity, by the way, is *not* due to bacterial decomposition; it results from the action of the *air* on the unsaturates in the oil.

Unsaturated oils are marvelous on the skin, softening it without leaving a greasy sensation at all, appearing to "penetrate" better than, say, mineral oil, which just sits on the surface and glares with a shiny look and feels greasy. Mineral oil is fine for a cleansing cream—where you *don't* want penetration—or for hair grooms where you *want* a sheen, but not for emollient creams or so-called "nourishing" creams.

SALICYLIC ACID—available at drug stores.

Salicylic acid is one of those old fashioned preservatives which used to be used quite commonly in cosmetics, but has now been supplanted by more powerful chemicals. These, however, are not generally available to the *home* cosmetic chemist. It is still used as a preservative for some food products, and of course, is the basis for the manufacture of a very famous drug called *acetyl*-salicylic acid (aspirin to you).

There are dermatological preparations on the market which take advantage of the "keratoplastic" (skin softening) action of this antiseptic, treating deep-down infections such as ringworm, or for removing corns and calluses. However, to get *that* kind of softening, you have to use such high percentages of salicylic acid that the preparation would be irritating if spread over a large area of skin.

For cosmetic use, we'll stick to the usual trace amounts needed for preservation of the product—about one-fourth teaspoon of the crystals per cup of cream or lotion. Always *dissolve* salicylic acid in the oil phase of your emulsion before making the cream. Do *not* simply add at the end, when the crystals will not dissolve.

SESAME OIL—available in some food stores and specialty health stores.

Sesame oil is a pale yellow, almost odorless, light weight oil which is much used for the manufacture of oleomargarine and cosmetics. It is often difficult to find in food stores, however.

Like safflower oil, sesame is quite unsaturated and penetrates the skin readily. It is an excellent skin emollient and softener. Its additional virtue is that it absorbs more *ultraviolet* light than any other natural oil. Ultraviolet is that part of the sunlight which includes the *burning rays.* Therefore, it makes a lot of sense to use this oil in suntan preparations, whose main purpose is to shield the skin from burning rays.

(By the way, did you know that *you can't get a sunburn through window glass,* no matter *how* long you sit in the sunlight which comes through it? The reason? Window glass is a "UV Absorber"—it absorbs the ultraviolet rays of sunlight, including that portion of the UV "spectrum" which burns the skin.)

SHAMPOO—at drug stores and supermarkets, department stores.

Most *clear* shampoos contain *lauryl sulfate* detergent, an excellent auxiliary emulsifier for making certain emulsions such as WATERLESS HAND CLEANER. Also, it can occasionally be substituted for 10 percent SOAP STOCK in some of the lotion formulas. However, since each shampoo on the market is likely to have slight variations in *its* formula, we could not generally base formulas on use of "clear shampoo." You *may* find that your favorite brand works wonders, however, replacing 10 percent SOAP STOCK in one of your favorite cosmetic recipes.

SHORTENING—at all food stores.

In this book, *shortening* always refers to *solid vegetable* shortening. Some oils are labelled "shortening oil" in food stores, and animal products such as lard and lard derivatives are also sold for the purpose. These are usable in cosmetics (as any fat or oil is) but will not give exactly the same product if used in a formula calling for the vegetable shortening.

Solid vegetable shortening is produced from liquid vegetable oils by a chemical process called *hydrogenation,* which solidifies them. Air is then whipped into it to give that creamy white consistency which is so familiar and makes it easy to measure out. Any odorless cooking grade is fine to use in cosmetics. Just try to get the *simplest* one (usually the cheapest!) *without* various magic additives such as silicones to prevent splattering, polyunsaturates, and other additives. Such additives *might* interfere with your emulsion, change it in some way.

Plain solid vegetable shortening contains *triglycerides,* solid fats which act as emulsion stabilizers and thickeners. That's why you're adding it to your cream.

SOAP FLAKES—pure soap flakes are available in the Soap and Detergents section of food stores, as well as in the baby products area of drug stores.

Formulas in this book which call for 10 percent SOAP STOCK will *not* work if you have not used *pure soap* to make up the stock base. Avoid all detergent flakes or mixtures of soap and detergents. Also, avoid all soap flakes with various miracle additives (bluing, softeners). Your best bet is to head for the baby products department and buy the smallest available box of those famous flakes which are guaranteed 99.44 percent pure soap.

Then make up the SOAP STOCK as directed, using one cup water for each ounce of soap flakes in the box. That way you'll be *sure* to have the exactly 10 percent solution required. Otherwise, soap flakes being so light and fluffy, it would be impossible to know exactly how much *weight* of soap you were measuring out if you did it by the cupful. If you use up the whole box of soap flakes, its label will state "Contents—7 oz. Av." or some such figure. In this particular case, you would dissolve the whole boxful in 7 cups of water and heat gently until they dissolve clearly.

SODIUM BENZOATE—available at drug stores on special request.

This is a commonly used food preservative. Is useful only in mildly *acidic* preparations, however, such as those products containing lemon juice. Will *not* preserve creams or lotions containing 10 percent SOAP STOCK, which is mildly alkaline.

STARCH—*see* CORNSTARCH

STEARIC ACID—available from candlemakers and soap makers, and from chemical supply houses.

Stearic acid is a crystalline white waxy material, a natural fatty acid present in tallow, in most vegetable oils, and in all animal fats. It is *the* major ingredient used in making bar soaps and many lubricants and candles contain it. A large proportion of cosmetic creams on the market today contain it also.

It gives pearliness to hand creams and that sort of firm consistency to creams which "gives" suddenly as you take a dab out of the jar, suddenly liquefying as you rub the cream onto your skin. A very *poor* substitute for it, which will work in some creams, is lard. Generally however, if you can't find a source of supply for it, don't attempt to make a cream calling for stearic acid.

TALC—available at all supermarkets and drug stores.

Talc is the softest mineral in the hardness scale (diamond is the hardest), existing as "platelets." Under the microscope it looks like a series of fish scales. These platelets *slide* across each other when you dust talc on your body as an after-bath powder. The softness and slipperiness of good quality talcs is something nothing else in the world can duplicate.

For this reason, talc is the basis for face powders, foot powders and powders for everything in between. It can also be added to face creams to give that added slip sensation. Generally, it is quite transparent and will not appear very white on the skin—unless a white pigment (such as zinc oxide) has been deliberately added to it.

TARRAGON—the dried leaves are available as an herb in most food stores.

The herb, tarragon (estragon) is used for flavoring soups, sauces, salad dressings and liqueurs. It is also used in perfumery for its "chypre" note. Home extracts can be successfully made by soaking the leaves in alcohol (ethanol) for about a week and then filtering the resulting green tincture. Such extracts make an excellent perfume for home cosmetics, but must *not* be used for flavoring food unless a drinkable alcohol (such as vodka) was used for the extract. Ethanol rubbing alcohol is *not* potable.

TEA—available at all food stores and specialty health shops.

Dried tea leaves, when extracted with boiling water in the normal manner of making the drink we call tea, give up their content of various *tannins* and *tannic acid*. Both of these compounds absorb that portion of sunlight (in the ultraviolet or UV portion) which burns the skin. Also, tannic acid itself happens to be very soothing to skin which has *been* burned, as many of you may already know from experience of applying wet tea compresses. In fact, drug stores also sell tannic acid jelly as a burn remedy.

Thus, since tea both helps to prevent and to soothe sunburn, how logical to base a suntan cream or lotion on the use of tea! The only problem is, tea does not contain too much of these chemicals, and therefore, even if you make quadruple strength tea as called for in the recipe, the result will be a suntan cream only about half as efficient as some of the better ones on the market today. It will give a fast tan and should not be depended on by those with *very* sensitive skins.

Note: *Instant tea* has had many of the tannins removed and is *only half as effective* as natural tea for this purpose.

Chamomile tea, available at specialized health food stores and some drug stores, contains azulene, a soothing ingredient which is most pleasant on the skin. Chamomile tea can be substituted for *water* in any emulsion where you would like to try the effect.

TINCTURE OF BENZOIN—available at most drug stores on request.

Benzoin is a natural balsamic resin exuded by certain trees growing in Thailand, Cambodia, Sumatra and Java. Tinctures of it (alcoholic solutions) are sold for use in vaporizers at home, to clear chest congestions.

It is also a preservative, a skin antiseptic and a perfumery ingredient. It forms astringent films on the skin.

TRAGACANTH—*see* GUM TRAGACANTH

VANILLA—the *bean* is available in specialty food shops; *extracts* are available in all food stores.

Vanilla extract is great in cosmetics as a perfume—either by itself or in mixtures. It is strong and sweet. Try it to round off a mixture of other extracts which you may have made and despaired of when the fragrance was not what you expected. A bit of vanilla added to such mixtures often smooths them out. Too much may sweeten your fragance more than you wish, however, so add it cautiously when compounding your own perfumes.

Note: Vanilla will turn some creams from a white to a light tan over a period of time. This is *not* spoilage, merely a natural discoloration due to one of the components of vanilla extract.

VEGETABLE COLORS—see FOOD COLORS

VEGETABLE JUICES—if you wish to use vegetable juices in your cosmetics, it is better to make them fresh as needed.

VEGETABLE SHORTENNG—see SHORTENING

VITAMINS—available in drug stores, some supermarkets.

Vitamins A and D are the only ones of real value in preparations for the skin. Buy the liquid (oily) type and add as part of the *oil phase* of emulsions. Use about one-fourth teaspoon per cup of cream or lotion. Can also buy *wheat germ oil with vitamins* A and D as a pet food supplement, but the vitamin content is pretty low here and the cod-liver oil odor difficult to mask. Use one teaspoon per cup of cream if you wish to try this mixture.

WHEAT GERM OIL—available at many drug stores and supermarkets.

Contains about 80 percent unsaturated fatty acids plus vitamin E. Has been recommended for cosmetic use. A rather exotic and expensive way to obtain benefits of poly-unsaturates on the skin.

WINTERGREEN—see METHYL SALICYLATE

WITCH HAZEL—available at all drug stores and some supermarkets as the *extract*.

Witch Hazel extract is mildly alcoholic, mildly astringent, a lovely soothing concoction obtained from twigs of the spotted alder bush which grows profusely in New England. You may occasionally hear of it under the Latin name *hamamelis* extract.

The astringency is due to the presence of some *tannins* (see discussion under TEA) and the fragrance of witch hazel is quite delightful. Has occasionally been used by itself as an after shave.

ZINC OXIDE—The *USP powder* is available at some drug stores. Do NOT use any other grade, such as may be available in paint and hobby shops.

Zinc oxide is a creamy white pigment with rather good covering power when used in face powders and liquid make-ups. It sticks to the skin rather tenaciously and is mildly antiseptic, mildly astringent, and—on the whole—rather soothing to irritations. This is why calomine lotion contains 8 percent zinc oxide.

The USP (pharmaceutical) grade is certified to be free of impurities such as lead and arsenic. Paint grades may contain traces of such, which of course should not be used in any cosmetic.

LIST OF TOOLS

A complete description of suggested tools for the cosmeticook is given in chapter two, Tools of the Trade.

> one or two eyedroppers
> one or two thin blade spatulas
> a three-speed electric hand beater
> set of metal measuring spoons
> one or two inexpensive enamel pots
> one or two Pyrex measuring cups
> containers, preferably with caps
> labels
> wide, low pan
> small funnel or bulb baster

WEIGHTS AND MEASURES

Naturally, everybody knows how many teaspoons are in a tablespoon, and how many ounces in a cup, and so forth. Nevertheless, when the chips are down and the emulsion is running and you're using only *half* the recipe quantities for everything because *that's* the size jar you have available to put it in—that's when it's convenient to have a handy reference table, just to make sure you're putting in *exactly* the right amount of each ingredient.

BASIC MEASURES
60 drops = 1 teaspoon (tsp.)
3 tsp. = 1 tablespoon (tbsp.)
2 tbsp. = 1 fluid ounce (fl. oz.)
8 fl. oz. = 1 cup (c.) = 16 tbsp.
2 cups = 1 pint = 16 fl. oz.
2 pints = 1 quart = 32 fl. oz.

10% SOLUTIONS
To make a 10% solution add one cup water for each *oz. Av.* of material to be dissolved.

TABLE OF EQUIVALENTS
1 fl. oz. = ⅛th cup = 2 tbsp. (= 6 tsp.)
2 fl. oz. = ¼th cup = 4 tbsp.
3 fl. oz. = ⅜th cup = 6 tbsp.
4 fl. oz. = ½ cup = 8 tbsp.
5 fl. oz. = ⅝th cup = 10 tbsp.
6 fl. oz. = ¾th cup = 12 tbsp.
7 fl. oz. = ⅞th cup = 14 tbsp.
8 fl. oz. = one cup = 16 tbsp.

INDEX

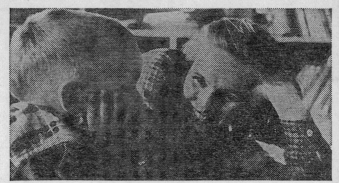

Today they're playing word games.
Before he's five, he can be reading 150 words a minute.

HOW TO GIVE YOUR CHILD A SUPERIOR MIND

A remarkable new book tells how you, yourself—at home—with no special training can actually add as much as thirty points to your child's effective I.Q....how you can help him move ahead quickly in school and enable him to be more successful in an education-conscious world.

Best of all, your child can achieve this early success without being pushed and without interference with a happy, normal, well-adjusted childhood.

GIVE YOUR CHILD A SUPERIOR MIND provides a planned program of home instruction that any parent can start using immediately. *You will learn:*

1. How to awaken your child's inborn desire to learn.
2. How to teach your child to read.
3. How to help your child streak ahead in math.
4. How to give your child the power of abstract reasoning.
5. How to increase your child's effective I.Q.

At all bookstores, or mail coupon today.➤

77278